The Integrative Helper

CONVERGENCE OF EASTERN
AND WESTERN TRADITIONS

WILLIAM L. MIKULAS
University of West Florida

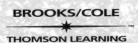

BROOKS/COLE

THOMSON LEARNING

Australia • Canada • Mexico • Singapore • Spain • United Kingdom • United States

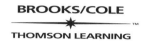

BROOKS/COLE

™

THOMSON LEARNING

Executive Editor: *Lisa Gebo*
Assistant Editor: *Alma Dea Michelena*
Marketing Team: *Caroline Concille, Megan Hansen, and Laura Hubrich*
Editorial Assistant: *Sheila Walsh*
Project Editor: *Mary Anne Shahidi*
Production Service: *Shepherd Inc.*
Manuscript Editor: *Patterson Lamb*

Permissions Editor: *Sue Ewing*
Interior Design: *Adriane Bosworth*
Cover Design: *Roger Knox*
Print Buyer: *Jessica Reed*
Typesetting: *Shepherd Inc.*
Printing and Binding: *Transcontinental Printing*

For more information about this or any other Brooks/Cole products, contact:
BROOKS/COLE
511 Forest Lodge Road
Pacific Grove, CA 93950 USA
www.brookscole.com
1-800-423-0563 (Thomson Learning Academic Resource Center)

For permission to use material from this work, contact us by
www.thomsonrights.com
fax: 1-800-730-2215
phone: 1-800-730-2214

Printed in Canada

10 9 8 7 6 5 4 3 2 1

Library of Congress Cataloging-in-Publication Data

Mikulas, William, L.
   The integrative helper : convergence of Eastern and Western traditions /
   William L. Mikulas.
      p. cm.
Includes bibliographical references and index.
ISBN 0-543-52517-2 (alk. paper)
1. Cross-cultural counseling. 2. Psychotherapy—Cross-cultral studies. I.Title.

BF637.C6 M524 2001
150—dc21   2001043583

*For Benita, a fountain of joy, nourishment,
and love at all levels of being*

Contents

Part Two

BIOLOGICAL LEVEL   29

Chapter 3

Biological Variables   31

Chapter 4

Biobehavioral Therapy   45

Part Three

BEHAVIORAL LEVEL   65

Chapter 5

Behavior   67

Chapter 6

Behavior Modification   77

Chapter 7

Behaviors of the Mind   85

Part Four

PERSONAL LEVEL   109

Chapter 8

Conscious Personal Reality   111

Chapter 9

Self and Will   128

Part Five

TRANSPERSONAL LEVEL   153

Chapter 10

The Transpersonal Domain   155

Chapter 11

The Way Beyond   166

Part Six

ACROSS LEVELS   177

Chapter 12

Integration and Themes   179

Preface

There are four interrelated objectives for this book:

1. To provide a readable, practical overview of the fundamental dynamics of human behavior and consciousness.
2. To highlight important contributions from the world's psychologies that are not well known in Western psychology.
3. To help readers develop their own integrated understanding of psychology and helping processes.
4. To identify knowledge and skills that an optimal psychologist or helper would have.

Chapter 1 elaborates on these objectives. And at the end of this preface is a listing of some of the helper skills, reader/client activities, and clinical examples found in the text. Next, I say a little more about for whom the book is intended, and then thank people who helped in its creation.

As stated in Chapter 1, this book is for anyone who functions as a helper with himself or herself and others, including psychologists, psychiatrists, social workers, counselors, teachers, parents, and others. The book is intended for use in college courses and for people in the field.

In terms of college courses, due to its broad and exploratory approach, the book could be a supplementary text in courses on therapy and change techniques in psychology, counseling, social work, and health. This is particularly true for instructors who wish to add one or more of the following components to their courses: powerful therapies from Asian psychologies that are coming into Western psychology, complementary psychophysical health practices that are being established by research and more and more supported by insurance companies and managed health care, important and widespread biological and transpersonal influences on psychology, and cross-cultural integrative models of psychology and change processes.

There are also courses for which this would be a primary text, such as courses specifically geared toward having students synthesize their knowledge and develop their own broad integrated perspectives. This includes senior honors courses and other undergraduate or graduate capstone courses. The book encourages students to integrate what they know and provides some possible conceptualizations for this integration. It also exposes them to many ideas and practices they have not yet considered. This can help them reflect on some of their assumptions and gain a more accurate understanding of their current knowledge and skills.

Currently, perhaps the most important and influential movement in clinical psychology and counseling is the development of integrative/eclectic therapies. Every year more and more courses are devoted to this topic, nationally and worldwide. This book is intended for such courses and covers many topics not found in any other such book. It would package very well with Gold's (1996) summary of Western psychotherapy integration and/or Wilber's (2000) overview of his Integral Psychology. Other possible readings are listed at the beginning of Chapter 2.

In addition to college courses, the book is intended for helpers in the field. After a necessarily limited formal education, such people continue to learn and grow through means such as personal reading, workshops, and professional experiences. This book contains many topics and change approaches that were not part of most of the helper's formal education, but which they may now be gradually encountering, such as some of the material from Eastern psychologies, biological psychology, and transpersonal psychology. This book provides a practical discussion of these topics, plus key references for further learning.

ACKNOWLEDGMENTS

Many people contributed to the development of this book. Jay Gould sharpened my biological discussion, Roz Hussong expanded my knowledge of cultural variables, and John Ritchie kept me abreast of important issues in men's psychology and the men's movement. John, and the students in my Conjunctive Psychology courses of fall 1998 and fall 2000, read through an entire earlier draft of the book and provided many helpful suggestions. The second conjunctive course also helped generate 49 of the 165 thought questions.

Special thanks go to my friend and production assistant Connie Works who delights in contributing to my books and papers. Because of her, I can write in longhand and later have all the advantages of computer technology. I marvel at her ability to type very quickly while also reading content. In addition to appreciating her great help in producing publications, I greatly value the person Connie, a quality lady of quiet strength who has made many people's lives better.

William L. Mikulas

PUBLISHER'S ACKNOWLEDGMENTS

The publisher wishes to thank the following manuscript reviewers: Elliott Ingersoll, Cleveland State University; Jackie Leibsohn, Seattle University; Sadye Logan, University of South Carolina; Stephen Marson, University of North Carolina-Pembroke; Ed Neukrug, Old Dominion University; Deane Shapiro, University of California, Irvine; Dale Smith, Western Kentucky University; and Timothy Walter, Oakland Community College.

Skills, Activities, and Examples Discussed in the Book

Helper Skills

mindfulness of breathing
relaxation procedures
mindfulness of body
seeing operant contingencies
seeing operant/respondent
   interrelationships

mindfulness of behavior
behavior modification
behaviors of mind
art of living

Reader/Client Activities

mindfulness of breathing
dependent origination
attachment log
mandala
personal tarot
self-meditations

pie exercise
loving-kindness meditation
journal keeping
right speech
conjunctive pyramid

Clinical Examples

Caucasian and Chinese
   assessment
food allergy
physical size
school anxiety
cognition and emotion

depth perception
teaching story
learning without awareness
expectation and perception
multiple selves

one

OVERVIEW

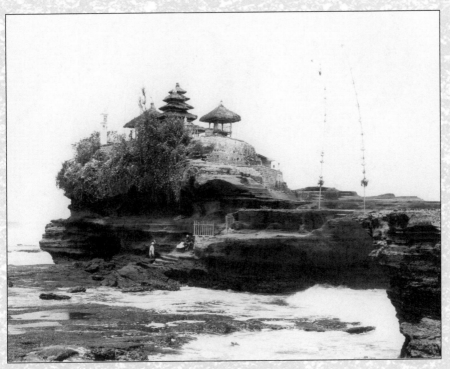

Photo by Benita Mikulas

BACKGROUND

What are the most important things that happened in the culture of the United States in the last half of the twentieth century? This is a question I have posed to many groups. The most common answer is related to computer technology (e.g., microchips, Internet). This is a good answer, as computer technology has certainly had strong effects on the culture, from very desirable to very problematic.

A second answer is the influx of Eastern thought, such as Indian yoga, Buddhist meditation, and Chinese acupuncture. Fifty years ago if I had wanted to learn about Tibetan dream yoga, I would probably have had to travel to Tibet, hire a guide and translator, and trek through the Himalayas in search of a teacher who would be willing to instruct me. Now I can sit at a computer in my office and order English translations of Tibetan dream yoga texts, and they will be delivered to me in a few days. Eastern influences now permeate many aspects of Western culture, including art, music, philosophy, religion, cuisine, economics, and ecology. Tibet's Dalai Lama is currently a best-selling author and celebrity as well as a great leader. And, most readers of this book have had some experience with an Eastern-based practice, such as yoga, meditation, tai chi, chi kung, or martial arts.

The influence of Eastern thought on Western psychology is particularly significant and important. Western psychologies of the near future will be very different because of this input. Over the last few decades, I have been heavily involved, as a practitioner, researcher, and teacher, in the interfacing of Eastern and Western psychologies. This book provides a general overview of the key concepts, practices, and references related to this exciting synthesis that is taking place around the world. I have been very fortunate in that I have done a lot of international traveling and living and am involved with many international groups concerned with the East-West integration. Hence, the ideas and practices discussed in this book represent what many people around the world are doing. All of this relates to one of the book's objectives: to highlight important contributions from the world's psychologies that are not well known in Western psychology.

A second objective for the text is to provide a readable, practical overview of the fundamental dynamics of human behavior and consciousness. Drawing from psychologies that have developed around the world, I survey our current knowledge of the important factors related to behavior change and personal growth. When I combine what we know from various sources, such as Western academic psychology, Buddhist psychology, and the yogic sciences, what are the universal constructs and dynamics that emerge, and how do they interrelate? The overview provided in this book is fairly general, as I am trying to develop a broad view and see interrelationships among disparate literatures and across the helping professions. Many key references are provided for the reader who wishes to pursue any topic in more detail. The overview is intended to be practical and readable. I want to consider the topics in clear, simple, logical language with an emphasis on their practical implications.

A primary audience for this book is students and practitioners trained in traditional Western academic programs. For these people, a little more in definitions and descriptions is provided from less-familiar literatures (e.g., ayurveda, pranayama, chi kung, dukkha, transpersonal).

Relatedly, names and schools of psychology well known to Western psychologists will occasionally be mentioned without definition. If readers are unfamiliar with one of these names or terms, this should not affect their understanding of the main points or facts.

HEURISTIC

The word "heuristic" is important in this book. It means stimulating interest and investigation, encouraging one to discover for oneself. Many of the examples and conceptual models were chosen for their heuristic value, as opposed to their academic trendiness or philosophical sophistication. Some examples, such as the Eastern metaphor of the mind as a drunken monkey, have established their heuristic value over thousands of years and across diverse cultures. Other examples are ones I have developed over decades of courses and workshops with many different types of people.

The intent of this book is to stimulate thought, not promote some theory or model. Readers should freely alter any of the conceptualizations to make them more personally heuristic. For example, I have found the four levels of being, introduced in the next chapter, to be very heuristic. But some readers may find it more heuristic to add another level or two. There is no problem here.

INTEGRATION

A third objective for the book is to help readers develop their own integrated understanding of psychology and helping processes. The text will provide a practical integration of the topics covered, suggesting general principles, causal relationships, sequential development, and so on. The heuristic intent is to stimulate the reader to develop her or his own integrated perspective. At different points some readers may disagree with and/or be offended by some conclusion, interpretation, bias, or omission. At such times, please remember that the intent of the book is to stimulate thought, not to advocate a position. Also, some of the specifics are less important than the goal of cultivating a broader, more integrated under-standing of human behavior and consciousness. Throughout the book I could have added many qualifications, alternative models or explanations, discussions of the nature and quality of research evidence, and clearer distinctions between opinions and facts; but this is contrary to my objectives, and this type of information can be found in the references and the sources to which they lead.

Consider the common situation of many practicing American psychologists. During their academic studies, they are exposed to some specialized Western approaches at the expense of others. Later, through personal reading, workshops, and professional experiences, they often encounter a bewildering mass of psycho-logical theories and therapies. Many try to be eclectic and to develop a unique and personal approach, drawing from the various psychologies they have encountered. The aim is an approach that personally speaks to the psychologist and addresses the complexities of the clients' problems. But the theories and therapies that he or she is trying to combine are often contradictory and confusing. Is there a solution? Yes; the one I offer is to develop a broader integrated perspective in which these specific therapies and theories become special cases.

As an exercise in thinking about broad integrative approaches, consider two heuristic models: Patanjali's classic integration of the yogic sciences and Ken Wilber's contemporary "integral" theory.

PATANJALI

About 200 C.E. (Common Era), Patanjali combined the various yogic practices of the time into one integrated model called "classical yoga" or "raja yoga," "raja" meaning "royal" (Eliade, 1975; Prabhavananda & Isherwood, 1953). Although lit-tle is known about Patanjali, he "was obviously a yoga adept who also had a great head on his shoulders" (Feuerstein, 1998, p. 284). His model includes the eight limbs of yoga: yama, niyama, asana, pranayama, pratyahara, dharana, dhyana, and samadhi. These terms are not important here, but their meaning is.

Yama is abstention from evil conduct, particularly in the social domain. Niyama is virtuous conduct and self-restraint, particularly as they relate to the inner life. Together, they emphasize ordering one's life along moral and practical guidelines. This includes nonviolence, not stealing, avoiding sexual excess, non-possessiveness, truthfulness, cleanliness of body and mind, practices to perfect body and mind, contentment, and study of self and spiritual works.

Asana originally meant immobilization of the body for meditation. After Patanjali, the meaning evolved to include the various positions of hatha yoga, what most Americans think of as yoga. Pranayama is the control of breath and vital energy, as discussed in Chapter 4.

Pratyahara is withdrawal of the senses; dharana is concentration; and dhyana is absorption meditation. Together they include quieting the mind and developing concentration, as discussed Chapter 7.

And samadhi is union with the divine ground. The word "yoga" means "yoke" or "union," and the ultimate goal of yoga is union with the divine ground. This will be discussed in Chapters 10 and 11 in terms of uncovering the transpersonal level of being.

The point is that Patanjali, and yoga in general, recognizes the importance of working with body, mind, and spirit in order to optimize health and well-being, including psychological health. This is a central theme of this book. Patanjali also included a philosophical view (a dualistic metaphysics), which is not accepted by all yogis, but all yogis recognize the importance of the practices related to the eight limbs. Similarly with this book; emphasis is given to effective practices, which can be conceptualized and philosophized about in many different ways.

KEN WILBER

Ken Wilber burst onto the scene in 1977 with his influential book *The Spectrum of Consciousness*, a comprehensive developmental model of consciousness that integrates Eastern and Western psychologies and philosophies. This publication marked the beginning of a highly prolific career in which Wilber has been gradually developing a more and more comprehensive stage model of development that he has applied to individual development (1980), cultural development (1983), evolution of religion (1984), and psychology and therapy (2000). In addition to integrating Eastern and Western psychologies, philosophies, and religions, Wilber continually applies his model to more and more domains of knowledge, incorporating such topics as art, morals, science, medicine, politics, ecology, gender studies, historical development, postmodern thought, and business. A significant feature of Wilber's theories is the importance given to transpersonal stages of development, a topic discussed later in this book.

The most comprehensive statement of Wilber's theory is his book *Sex, Ecology, Spirituality* (1995). A more popular and readable version of this theory is his book *A Brief History of Everything* (1996a). One or both of these books are important reading for people interested in developmental psychology, transpersonal psychology, evolution, models of consciousness, or the interface of Eastern and Western philosophies. Wilber's theories have influenced many psychologists (e.g., Rowan, 1993; Vaughan, 1995). Particularly interesting is how different therapies may apply to different stages of psychospiritual development.

Wilber's theory is a stage model, based on and including classic stage theories such as those of Freud and Piaget. The assumption underlying stage models of human development is that people move through a fixed set of stages, which are the same for everyone and occur in the same order for everyone. Freud suggested that everyone goes through the same stages of psychosexual development, and Piaget argued similarly for cognitive development. Wilber postulates that each stage includes and surpasses previous stages.

The problem with stage models is that human development is not so simple and is often culturally influenced. Development is not a simple linear progression; there is movement back and forth and spiraling. People often seem to be at different stages depending on circumstances. And it is not clear that everyone must move through the same stages in the same order. Wilber's initial theory was very popular, partly because of its simplicity. But it suffered from many of the problems of other stage theories. Over time, Wilber altered his theory, making it more complex and more valid. The major change is the suggestion that there are about two dozen different, relatively independent, developmental "lines" (Wilber, 2000). Examples include cognitive, moral, interpersonal, affective, and spiritual lines. Wilber postulates that development along each line goes through the exact same sequence of potential stages, although not at the same rate. Thus, a person's overall development, a combination of many lines, may not show a simple linear and sequential development.

Another feature of Wilber's theory is the model of the "four quadrants," a scheme he uses to classify and integrate all knowledge. A number of topics in this book, *The Integrative Helper,* relate to Wilber's quadrants. The first quadrant is "interior-individual (intentional)," the domain of subjective consciousness and "I-language." Topics in this book that correspond to topics Wilber puts in this quadrant are breathwork, cognitive therapy, and mindfulness. The second quadrant is "exterior-individual (behavioral)," the domain of the brain and "it-language." Related topics in this book include nutrition, bodywork, and drugs.

The third quadrant is "interior-collective (cultural)," the domain of values, meaning, worldview, and "we-language." In this book it includes cultural differences and the interpersonal. The fourth quadrant is "exterior-collective (social)," the domain of social systems and "it-language." Topics in this book related to the fourth quadrant are the issue of environmental pollution and some gender-related social issues.

Wilber's position is that a comprehensive model of knowledge, and often a comprehensive plan for an individual's life, must take into account all four quadrants. In the context of this book, I would say that the integrative helper must consider possible interventions from all four quadrants.

In addition to the specifies of his theory, Wilber has brought clear and discriminating thinking to many important issues, particularly related to transpersonal development. Two important examples of Wilber's clarifying thinking are his delineating different types of knowing and his classic explanation of the pre-trans fallacy, both discussed in Chapter 10.

Despite his importance for some areas of psychology, Wilber is very rarely mentioned in mainstream American texts and journals. There are many reasons for this omission (not necessarily "good" reasons): Wilber is not a psychologist and has not had extensive formal education or training in psychology. He does not have an advanced degree and is not affiliated with any university or research center. He does not go to conventions or publish in mainstream journals. And he emphasizes the transpersonal, which is controversial.

Continuing to think about different aspects of integrative models, consider the similarities and differences between Wilber's approach to psychology, which he calls "Integral Psychology," and the approach of this book, called "Conjunctive Psychology." Both approaches are inclusive; all basic schools of psychology and forms of therapy are included. The question is not whether bodywork, behavior modification, psychoanalysis, or meditation is the one best form of treatment. Rather the question is when and where each of these different interventions is appropriate, and how they interact with each other. Conjunctive Psychology readily incorporates all of Integral Psychology; and all of the components of Conjunctive Psychology could be mapped into the four quadrants of Integral Psychology.

Both Conjunctive Psychology and Integral Psychology emphasize drawing from all the world's disciplines, with initial emphasis on the integration of Western and Asian psychologies. And both psychologies include recognition of the necessity and importance of including the transpersonal domain.

The major and most significant difference between the two psychologies is that Integral Psychology is philosophy and Conjunctive Psychology is applied psychology. Wilber is a philosopher, and his theory is based on his own reading, thinking, and meditating. Wilber's approach is not based on his own clinical experience and research. The major heuristic value of Wilber's work is philosophical, not applied. If professional helpers read Integral Psychology, they might not come away with practical ideas of things they can do the next day in the clinic, halfway house, classroom, or office. The ideals and views of Integral Psychology are exciting. What are their heuristic values relative to practice?

It must be emphasized that Wilber does not argue for philosophy over practice! In fact, he would strongly advocate the opposite. He continually says it is more important to practice meditation than to read his writings about meditation. It is just that Wilber is a philosopher, and his great contribution to our integrative understanding is his philosophical models. Of course, Wilber's writings do contain a number of practical hints, such as those related to meditation practice. Most important for the transpersonal practitioner is Wilber's continual and skillful pointing to the fundamental ground of consciousness.

Conjunctive Psychology is an applied psychology. My professional work over the last few decades has involved educating future and current professional helpers (e.g., psychologists, counselors, teachers, business people) in addition to my own personal clinical work. I am more interested in effective ways to help people change than in complex theory building. Whereas Wilber constructs beautiful maps of some territories, I am more interested in helping people learn practical ways to navigate through these territories, perhaps guided by a Wilber map. I expect everyone who reads this book to bring from it some new, significant, powerful, practical ideas to apply to his or her own work or self. The following is a small sample of possibilities: A teacher may decide to investigate the air quality of her classroom, as it may relate to health and behavior problems. A social worker may add a food diary to part of her assessment procedures for some clients. A parent may begin rewarding approximations to various social and educational behaviors as a way to increase a child's self-esteem. A clinical psychologist may learn to quiet her mind in order to be more empathic. Or a spiritual practitioner may realize her ego is trying to transcend itself, which cannot happen.

Wilber's developmental stage theory is central to Integral Psychology. When integrating psychologies, Wilber emphasizes those that are most relevant to his theory. In Conjunctive Psychology, developmental processes are valued, but they are not necessarily central. In Integral Psychology, the transpersonal applies only to the last stages of development, although people may have glimpses of the transpersonal at any stage. Conjunctive Psychology stresses that the transpersonal level of being is always, already present, something that Wilber points out often. Despite developmental processes that may move toward the transpersonal, in Conjunctive Psychology emphasis is given to working with all four levels of being now (biological, behavioral, personal, transpersonal). No level is more important than another, and they are totally intertwined. Transpersonal components of a change program have importance beyond their relation to the client's developmental stages.

As a result of differences such as those described earlier, the topics included and emphasized in Conjunctive Psychology are extremely different from those in Integral Psychology. Two of many examples include behavior modification and psychoanalysis. The field of behavior modification contains some of the most effective and most applicable procedures for changing behaviors, which is a significant part of what most professional helpers are involved with. Hence, behavior modification is an important part of Conjunctive Psychology (Chapters 5–7). However, behavior modification is largely irrelevant to Wilber. It is possible to map one type of behaviorism as a philosophy into one of Wilber's quadrants (e.g., exterior-individual), but behavior modification has much of great value to contribute to all four quadrants. Also, one might map certain behavior modification strategies into certain developmental stages, but behavior modification is usually useful and appropriate at almost all developmental stages.

Because Wilber's theory draws from and incorporates Freudian theory, Wilber assumes the widespread applicability of psychoanalysis, and he advocates therapies with similar approaches. It is probably the case, however, that psychoanalysis is not as applicable or effective as Wilber assumes, and there may often be more effective forms of therapy. The fact that psychoanalysis logically follows from integral theory does not mean that it is necessarily effective in a particular real-world situation. Psychoanalytic approaches are highly valued in Conjunctive Psychology but in a more restricted sense than in Integral Psychology.

Integral Psychology and Conjunctive Psychology are very different in approach, objectives, and what each emphasize. They are not in conflict; they supplement and complement each other and they each include each other. By reflecting on the similarities and differences outlined here, readers can better decide what aspects and objectives they might want for their own personal integrative approach. Also, they may begin considering issues and problems in developing integrated models. And, hopefully, the above discussion will help readers to have more accurate expectations for this book.

For people who wish to learn more about Wilber's thinking, *Integral Psychology* (2000) is an excellent complement to this book, and *Eye to Eye* (1996b) is a good introduction to some of his more general thinking. Washburn (e.g., 1995) provides an alternative developmental model that covers much of the same ground as Wilber but makes very different assumptions.

CONJUNCTIVE PSYCHOLOGY

Years ago, I was at a national convention of behavior therapy where I had presented a paper and a student of mine had presented a research study. A colleague approached me and complemented me on "nice data," but was concerned that I was involved with Buddhism and other such "airy-fairy" stuff. Later, I was sitting around with Ram Dass, a popular Western yogi and previous Harvard psychologist (formerly Richard Alpert). Ram Dass was excited that I had a formal course in Buddhist psychology, but he wondered why I was also involved with behavior modification. "Aren't we past behaviorism now?" he asked.

Well, I knew that behavior modification is very powerful and useful, as is Buddhist psychology, and meditation, and . . . What did not exist was a broad enough conceptual framework to encompass them all. So I made up Conjunctive Psychology, where behavior modification and Buddhism can both be "true" and valid (e.g., Mikulas, 1995, 1996b). To be accurate, I should note that since the early days of behavior modification, some people have been interested in its intersection with Buddhism (e.g., Padmal de Silva, Alan Marlatt, Deane Shapiro). And Ram Dass would readily admit the importance of behavior modification to help clear the way for spiritual progress.

Conjunctive psychology is more an approach than a theory. It is an approach with three premises: (1) The most useful and powerful psychology can be developed with greatest efficiency by drawing from the wealth of psychological knowledge that exists worldwide. This does not mean indiscriminately accepting something because it is yogic or Buddhist, or rejecting something because it comes from another culture. Such an eclectic undertaking involves using clear thinking and testing ideas experientially and experimentally. (2) Ideas and interventions from all levels of being, including the transpersonal, must be considered if one is to have a comprehensive and effective psychology. How and why the transpersonal is included is discussed later in this book (Chapters 10 and 11). (3) Emphasis must be given to developing a practical, integrated model that includes interactions across levels. This is a basic objective for this book.

Anyone who agrees with these three premises may say his or her orientation is that of Conjunctive Psychology. (This has nothing to do with credentials, degrees, licensing, or membership in a formal organization.) Many people now, nationally and internationally, call themselves Conjunctive Psychologists in addition to, not instead of, whatever else they are. It is simply a shortcut way to identify some common interests.

This is the orientation taken in this text. As you read please always remember that the summaries, opinions, models, and speculations in this book are just my current version of "Conjunctive Psychology." Thus, nothing is offered as "true," but only as the working position of Conjunctive Psychology. Definitions are not necessarily universally accepted, but only the way the terms are used in Conjunctive Psychology. Conceptual models are not the "right" way to think, but only a way that has proven heuristic in Conjunctive Psychology. Conjunctive Psychology is more an approach than a theory, although it embraces many theoretical speculations and stances. The next chapter will elaborate on this psychology.

INTEGRATIVE HELPER

The fourth objective for this book is to identify knowledge and skills that an optimal psychologist or helper would have. In this book, the term "helper" is used in the broadest sense to include anyone who functions as a psychological adviser with

himself or herself, and with others. This includes psychologists, psychiatrists, social workers, counselors, parents, teachers, and anyone acting in a helping capacity. The term "helper" is used because it basically is a more general term than alternatives such as "therapist," "psychologist," or "change agent." It refers to a person who provides informed and practical advice. Readers may replace the term "helper" in this book with any preferred term, such as "adviser," "teacher," "parent," "therapist," "psychologist," or "conjunctive psychologist."

The "integrative helper" is the ideal helper in the broad, integrated view. One need not be an authority on the many topics covered in this book, but the integrative helper must have some basic understanding of these topics and how they relate to his or her domains of interest and clients. The integrative helper must realize what he or she knows and does not know and when to refer clients to others for assessment and/or treatment. Throughout the book are examples of conceptual knowledge and experiential skills that the integrative helper should consider cultivating. Some of these are listed at the end of the preface.

SUMMARY

American psychology is currently in a state of great change. One reason is the dramatic influx of theories and practices from other world psychologies, particularly Asian psychologies. A second reason is the demand from practitioners and clients for a more holistic and integrated approach to psychology and health. This book provides an overview of some of these changes, highlighting topics not yet well known.

The term "Conjunctive Psychology" is used to describe the general approach of gradually developing a practical and heuristic integration of the world's knowledge about behavior and consciousness. An "integrated helper" is a person who uses such an approach to help himself or herself and others. This helper might be a psychologist, counselor, social worker, health adviser, teacher, parent, or someone else.

Two examples of integrative holistic approaches include the works of Patanjali and Wilber. Patanjali synthesized the various yoga schools of his time into a classic and influential model that emphasizes body, mind, and spirit in one's overall health and personal/spiritual growth. Wilber provides a contemporary philosophical model that includes four quadrants for classifying everything.

AUTHOR'S REFLECTIONS

Wilber's work is controversial for many reasons, such as what he does and does not include. Some criticize his theory because of what he omits or does not emphasize, such as my comments about behavior modification. Others object to what he does include, such as the transpersonal. Similarly for Conjunctive Psychology, some will object to what is not included or emphasized; others will object to what is included. For example, among the reviewers of an earlier draft of this book, a couple became very angry because I suggested there might be deficiencies in Western psychology that could be helped with practices from Eastern psychologies.

Some people are very threatened by what they do not know. I have recommended Wilber's work to many developmental psychologists, and a couple were very disturbed by this suggestion. They considered themselves experts in developmental psychology; yet here was a body of work purported to be important for developmental psychology, and they knew nothing about it. Rather than being interested and delighted, they were threatened and became aggressive. Many people will be threatened by some of the ideas in this book, simply because the ideas are new to them. Of course, new does not mean true, better, useful, or anything else. And there are lots of other reasons for disagreeing with things in this book.

Textbook publishers are usually not interested in books that are on the leading edge of the field. They want books whose content will be very familiar and comfortable to the instructor. One psychology editor told me that her publisher wanted texts that are about five years behind the field.

If you, the reader, are using this book as a text in a class, you are very lucky, for your instructor is probably not threatened by the unknown or by the inevitable changes in the field. He or she may even be involved in some of these new areas. But you must realize that your instructor cannot be knowledgeable of all the topics mentioned in this book. He or she will not be a traditional instructor using a traditional text. Rather, the instructor and you with your fellow students will be traveling together, all with contributions to make. The purpose of this book is simply to be heuristic, suggesting some literatures and practices that may warrant your investigation. Key references are provided for further exploration. The first step is to consider some of the aspects of Conjunctive Psychology in a little more detail, as I do in the next chapter.

THOUGHT QUESTIONS

At the end of each chapter is a set of thought questions. Their purpose is to help readers reflect on, understand, and integrate ideas of the chapter. The questions vary on many dimensions, including breadth, difficulty, and time to answer. An excellent thought question is to make up a thought question. I did this with a class in Conjunctive Psychology and some of the class members' thought questions are included in this text, designated by parentheses around the question number. If any of you have good thought questions, please send them to me via the publisher. Add a signed statement that allows me to use your questions.

1. If you were to develop an integrated model of psychology, what properties would you want this model to have?
2. Construct a 2×2 matrix based on Wilber's four quadrants. What aspects of your personal practices and/or vocation fit into the four different quadrants? What are the implications of your answer?

GENERAL APROACH

The history of Western thought has generally been one of fractionalization and specialization. Religion and science battle and carve out their own domains. Science breaks into many separate disciplines, which develop their own terminology and programs. Psychology separates from philosophy and divides into two feuding camps: experimentalists and clinicians. Clinical psychology gradually disintegrates into a mass of contradictory theories and therapies. Academicians reward themselves for very specialized research and thinking.

But for the practicing helper, things are not so simple. An overspecialized theory that generates clean research is not necessarily useful in dealing with the complexities of the client's concerns. The integrative helper needs a broader model to work from. Gradually, many in the clinical field became dissatisfied with the fractionated and overspecialized state of the field and sought more powerful therapeutic models by combining different approaches.

INTEGRATION

By the mid-1980s, the movement toward integrating therapeutic approaches was becoming a major force in Western psychology (Gold, 1996; Goldfried, 1982; Mahoney, 1991; Mahrer, 1989; Norcross & Goldfried, 1992; Prochaska & Di-Clemente, 1984; Staats, 1996; Stricker & Gold, 1993). Very slowly people began piecing psychology back together and embedding it in related disciplines.

Two outside forces had a strong influence on the development of integrative models. The first was the demand by consumers for more "holistic" approaches to health and healing. People in the United States now spend more on complementary approaches to health (e.g., yoga, acupuncture, meditation) than on traditional medicine (e.g., drugs and surgery). The second force was the influx of Eastern psychologies, discussed below.

Examples of pieces of the integration include combinations of psychoanalysis and behavior modification (Arkowitz & Messer, 1984; Wachtel, 1977), behavior modification and Buddhism (de Silva, 1984, 1985; Mikulas 1978b, 1981), and Buddhism and psychoanalysis (Brazier, 1995; Epstein, 1995; Fromm, et al., 1960; Suler, 1993).

NAMAP

By "Western psychologies" I mean the primary psychologies of Western Europe, the Americas, and academically related countries. Within the Western psychologies the group that has been dominant is called here NAMAP (North American mainstream academic psychology). NAMAP theories, approaches to research, journals, and texts command the Western field. Almost all introductory psychology texts provide the same collections of NAMAP theories, assumptions, and research findings. A person with a psychology degree from a major American university will have almost exclusively learned this mainstream psychology.

The "North American" part of NAMAP recognizes that European psychologies are different from the psychologies of the United States and Canada, and South American psychologies are even more different. The "mainstream academic" component recognizes that NAMAP is often quite different from the psychologies of the practicing therapist and the "new" psychologies developing outside of NAMAP.

Throughout this book, NAMAP will be a strawperson, partially for the sake of the following objective: to highlight important contributions from the world's psychologies that are not well known in Western psychology. Like all other world psychologies, NAMAP has its own set of assumptions, beliefs, and limitations, which are often driven by political/social/psychological forces. As many readers have been educated within NAMAP, some of its limitations and biases will periodically be pointed out. This is not to criticize or attack NAMAP, but to facilitate developing a broader, more integrated understanding. Of course, all statements made about NAMAP are generalizations, and thus there are many exceptions and qualifications, as can be found in references throughout this book.

For example, two important limitations of NAMAP relate to development and religion. Historically, when students explored human development within this context, they got the impression that most or all major development was over by early adulthood, a view encouraged by Freud and Piaget (Erikson and Levinson are exceptions). By the 1990s, NAMAP views had begun to reflect the awareness that developmental issues related to the bulk of a person's life had been overlooked, and the idea of life-span developmental models gained popularity. But what are still conspicuously missing are discussion, theories, and research related to later stages of adult development, including transpersonal domains (cf. Alexander & Langer, 1990; Wade, 1996; Washburn, 1995; Wilber, 1995, 2000).

Many NAMAP clients of mainstream psychology in the second half of their lives encounter serious mid-life, existential, or spiritual crises. What NAMAP needs, and doesn't have, is a comprehensive developmental model that provides guidelines for the integrative helper to assist clients in continuing their personal growth. To optimally help clients discover happiness, peace of mind, fulfillment, and liberation requires understanding of transpersonal levels of development.

The second limitation of NAMAP is its approach to religion. In the United States, 60 percent of the people feel that religion is "very important" in their lives (Gallup, 1995), and clients in therapy consider it appropriate to discuss religious and spiritual concerns (Rose et al., 2001). But historically, in NAMAP's quest to be "scientific," it has actively excluded religion. Some prestigious psychology departments are noted for not allowing reference to religion, except in a derogatory sense. Some academic psychologists have been denied tenure because their research included religious variables. Therapists trained in NAMAP generally receive no education on how to include the client's religious beliefs and spiritual practices in the assessment and treatment program. In one survey, 83% of psychologists reported that religious and spiritual issues were never or rarely included in their training, although 54% desired such training (Shafranske & Malony, 1990). Counselors trained in counseling programs are more likely to be exposed to the importance of religious and spiritual factors (e.g., Hinterkopf, 1997; Ingersoll, 1997), and the field of social work is giving more and more attention to the spiritual needs of clients (e.g., Canada, 1988).

Heavily influenced by Freud, psychiatrists and psychologists often see religious beliefs as a sign of mental illness. An important example of this is the American Psychiatric Association's *Diagnostic and Statistical Manual of Mental Disorders* (*DSM*). The *DSM* is the main system that psychiatrists, psychologists, and others use in classifying people. In this system, religious beliefs and spiritual experiences are generally seen as signs of psychopathology. In version IV of the *DSM*, a minor category was added that includes "distressing experiences that involve loss or questioning of faith, problems associated with conversion to a new faith, or questioning of spiritual values that may not necessarily be related to an organized church or religious institution." This inclusion is a significant step forward for NAMAP, but it is still a very small part of what must ultimately be considered.

Conjunctive Psychology recognizes that the client's religious and spiritual beliefs and practices may be very important to the client and may be related to the clinical problems and/or their treatment. Assessment must include how these beliefs and practices help and/or harm the client. In most cases, we need to work within the constraints and strengths of the client's beliefs and practices. Perhaps the spiritual practices can be packaged with other treatment components. For example, behavior modification, which is relatively culture free, can be done within the context of Buddhism (Mikulas, 1981, 1983b) or the Judeo-Christian tradition (Lasure & Mikulas, 1996). In some cases, it may be ethically and practically appropriate to challenge some of the beliefs. It should be noted that within NAMAP there is a gradual awakening to the importance of including religious variables, sometimes in the context of cultural diversity (Bergin, 1991; Emmons, 1999; Kelly, 1995; Shafranske, 1996; Worthington et al., 1996). Furthermore, one of the divisions of the American Psychological Association focuses on religious issues.

EASTERN PSYCHOLOGIES

By "Eastern psychologies" I mean the predominantly Asian psychologies that have been heavily influenced by Indian and Chinese yoga, Buddhism, and Taoism. Although Eastern thought has been coming into the West for thousands of years, geographical distances, language differences, and cultural biases greatly limited

Westerners' knowledge of Eastern psychologies. When Jung became interested in Eastern thought, there was little information available for him; hence, he developed some misconceptions (Coward, 1985).

But beginning in the second half of the 20th century, things changed dramatically. Wars, the Peace Corps, spiritual seeking, and international trade brought Westerners to the East and Easterners to the West. Soon there were English translations of many previously inaccessible Eastern works. Eastern concepts, such as Zen, began appearing widely. There are now books relating Zen Buddhism to seeing, listening, running, writing, eating, archery, baseball, skiing, golf, mountain climbing, programming, career planning, management, sex, fatherhood, being black, time, depression, addiction recovery, bridge, guitar, pottery, driving, motorcycles, and studying. Quite probably, the influx of Eastern thought is one of the most significant factors in Western 20th century history. As a result, there is now a sizable literature comparing and combining Eastern and Western psychologies, which was an important source for this book (Kwee, 1990; Mikulas, 1991; Sheikh & Sheikh, 1996).

Eastern bodies of knowledge are much more integrated than are Western ones. Psychology is intertwined with biology, sociology, and religion. In traditional Asian cultures, there is no word or role for a psychologist. In these cultures it makes no sense to treat a person's mind as separate from other concerns, such as nutrition, energy, family relations, and spiritual practices. For example, ayurveda (ayu = life, veda = knowledge) is the natural healing system of India, developed over thousands of years. It includes working with nutrition, herbs, energy, color, massage, yoga, meditation, psychology, lifestyle, spirituality, and surgery. One must deal with body, mind, and spirit. On the one hand, the integrated nature of Eastern thought provides Westerners many ideas about developing an integrated model of healing in general and psychology in specific. On the other hand, it has been difficult for Westerners to abstract from Eastern thought what would be considered specifically psychological.

In the United States, the Eastern/Western distinction can be seen in the approach to yoga and martial arts. For most people in the United States, "martial arts" refers to a form of fighting and "yoga" is primarily stretching exercises. This is because we have extracted from the Asian systems one specialized component. But in the traditional Asian approaches, martial arts is a complete system of health, healing, energy, meditation, spirituality, and often massage. The fighting forms are a small part. And yoga, in its broadest sense, includes body postures, energy, breathing, nutrition, meditation, spiritual practices, and ethics (Feuerstein, 1998).

Despite widespread Western interest in Eastern thought and the probable significant impact of Eastern psychologies, there is little or no mention of Eastern contributions to psychology in most of NAMAP's curricula, courses, journals, or texts. One reason is that the Eastern literature is relatively new to NAMAP and Eastern psychological theories and data are buried in unfamiliar forms. A second reason is that because psychology is intertwined with spirituality in Eastern systems, it is all considered religion by NAMAP, and therefore irrelevant and/or inappropriate. A third reason is NAMAP's determination to consider only evidence that has been established by contemporary Western research methods. NAMAP intentionally ignores massive bodies of data that have been collected over thousands of years and across very diverse cultures. Thus, it is gradually rediscovering things that have long been well known in the world's psychologies. A dramatic example of this is in the fields of cognitive therapy and cognitive behavior therapy, where NAMAP researchers/theorists have struggled fairly unsuccessfully with basic issues of mental control, such as the problems related to intrusive/undesirable thoughts. How to develop mental control is one of the strengths of the Eastern psychologies, as discussed later.

Comparisons of Eastern and Western psychologies have uncovered areas of overlap, ways in which they complement and expand on each other, and important challenges to the assumptions, models, and approaches of each. There are strengths and weaknesses to both the Western and Eastern approaches, but an integration of the two can resolve most of the sources of weakness. The position of Conjunctive Psychology is that a comprehensive, integrated psychology must draw from all the world's major psychologies for efficiency of development, among other reasons. The working assumption is that it is possible to develop a psychology that is superordinate to both Western and Eastern psychologies and includes them as special cases. This book is a piece of the project. Note that not all the world's major psychologies are represented in this book. For example, the very rich African healing systems, which have many parallels with ayurveda, are not represented because I am not yet adequately knowledgeable of them.

CULTURAL DIFFERENCES

Drawing from the world's psychologies facilitates our appreciation and understanding of cultural differences. Cultures differ in their values, motivations, emotions, perceptions, family structure, child-rearing practices, personal time and space, relationship of the individual to the group, ways of doing business, and history. The field of cross-cultural psychology deals with these types of issues, including implications for counseling (Matsumoto, 1996; Pedersen et al., 1996; Ponterotto et al., 1995).

This is very important in the United States where over one-third of all Americans are nonwhite, and this proportion is growing. It is also important when the client is from another country or when we take an approach to therapy from one country into another country. Many NAMAP therapies are not applicable to cultures in other countries and may produce disastrous results. And many NAMAP personality theories and assessment devices are heavily culturally biased.

Integrative helpers are aware of the personal impact of their own cultures on themselves and the relativity of their own values, perceptions, and beliefs. Integrative helpers recognize the importance of understanding the client's culture and how cultural differences between client and helper may affect the helping process. Thus, when an African American integrative helper from Chicago moves to southern California, she or he will recognize the probable need to learn about Latino cultures.

The integrative helper cannot and need not be aware of all the differences among the many cultures. But the integrative helper needs to know the types of questions to ask when learning about cultural differences in general, and how they affect the helping process. What is the culture's understanding of "health?" How does the individual relate to the culture and how does this affect the sense of self? What types of pressures are there to conform to group norms? What are distinctive aspects of the culture's values, motives, and any sense of fatalism? What type of respect is there for parents? How do families and others in the culture use guilt and shame? What are important areas of self-control and hesitation (e.g., modesty, humility, patience, tolerance, and anger)? What are ways in which the client will express or present emotions, problems, and self? What are gender issues related to family, community, and the helper? What are different patterns and styles of communication and how are they embedded in various contexts? What are the history, current concerns, and legal issues of the culture? To what extent has the culture been incorporated into mainstream society? How much development has there been of a minority identity?

Therapeutic strategies are influenced by the culture. What are the client's expectations of help? How available is the helper expected to be at various times? How much need is there for structure and direction? What type of atmosphere is most conducive to good therapy? To what extent and how should the family be involved in the therapy? How appropriate, if at all, are approaches of self-disclosure and confrontation, and what form should they take?

The integrative helper learns about the culture by reading professional literature concerning the culture and literature from the culture (e.g., novels, biographies). As much as possible and practical, the helper gets involved with people and events in the community of the culture. The integrative helper appreciates this opportunity to become more aware of and transcend his or her own cultural assumptions and biases, while being comfortable with cultural differences. This facilitates the development of empathy—in this case, the ability to see, feel, and think, to some extent, from the point of view of another culture.

As an example, what constitutes appropriate assertive behavior varies tremendously between and within cultures. The average Thai woman could not be as socially initiating as the average American woman. What is considered being open and honest by American men might be seen as lacking subtlety by Chinese or as being boorish by Japanese. Maintaining eye contact is good in some white cultures; but in other cultures, it is disrespectful, rude, or aggressive (e.g., some Native American, African American, and Asian cultures). Common NAMAP therapeutic goals of individualism, independence, and assertiveness may be more appropriate with American men than women, would be in conflict with some Native American values, and are counter to the norms of more collectivist cultures, such as most Asian cultures.

A Western therapist might stress independence, assertiveness, nonconformity, competition, freedom, individual needs, expression of feelings, and self-actualization. An Eastern therapist might stress interdependence, compliance, conformity, cooperation, security, collective goals, control of feelings, and collective actualization (Ho, 1985). Caucasian and Chinese American therapists were asked to evaluate Caucasian and Chinese clients from videotaped interviews (Li-Repac, 1980). Caucasian therapists saw the Chinese clients as anxious, awkward, confused, nervous, and reserved; the Chinese therapists saw the same clients as adaptable, alert, ambitious, dependable, friendly, and practical. The Caucasian therapists saw the Caucasian clients as affectionate, adventurous, and easygoing, while the Chinese therapists saw the same clients as active, aggressive, and rebellious.

GENDER DIFFERENCES

Different "cultures" may be based on differences in age, physical strengths and limitations, socioeconomic status, religion, sexual preferences, or gender. In Conjunctive Psychology, we recognize that men and women come from different cultures. They differ in their perceptions, values, styles of communication, ways of expressing emotions, approaches to working and playing together, ways of building friendships, strategies of problem solving, and expectations of relationships (Gray, 1993; Moir & Jessel, 1991; Schaef, 1981; Tanenbaum, 1989; Tannen, 1990, 1994). To what extent gender differences are biologically based and/or learned is often difficult to determine and sometimes socially controversial. It unfortunately needs to be stressed that "different" does not mean unequal in a general sense, or better or worse, nor is it justification for social or economic discrimination. In the 1960s and 1970s in the United States, discussion or research on gender differences was generally a taboo topic, being falsely equated with sexism.

Consider some common differences between U.S. men and women, remembering that these are generalizations that certainly do not apply to all individuals to the same extent. In conversation, men are more concerned with conveying information, getting to the bottom line, problem solving, and maintaining their independence and position in the group. Women are more concerned with simply expressing feelings, playing with ideas, and using conversation to expand relationships and create connections and intimacy. At the end of a day a wife may like to talk about the details of the day as a way of strengthening the relationship, but the husband finds this somewhat boring, has had enough of the day's events, and sees conversation as a means to exchange information. Men will often take an oppositional stance, challenging and kidding the other person, particularly if the other person is a man. To them, refusing to argue might suggest you don't care. Women, on the other hand, often see no reason or advantage to such an approach. And thus they may be perceived by some men as being weaker. Silence often means to men that everything is fine, while to women it may mean something is wrong. A woman might nod and make sounds to show she is listening, while the man interprets this as showing agreement (Tannen, 1990, 1994).

Men's relationships develop side by side, while women's relationships develop face to face. A relationship between two women will often deepen as they talk to each other, exchanging details of each other's lives, including perceptions, concerns, and history. A relationship between two men may deepen when they do something together, such as play a game or sport, fix a car, go on an adventure, or fight a battle. Women often can't understand how men's friendships can develop with such little talking. Men often can't understand how women can enjoy such long, detailed, personal conversations. Men tend to have fewer same sex friends than women and often report being less close to friends.

Men will often see the individual as subordinate to the group and will be willing to sacrifice the individual for the good of the team (e.g., sports team, business, war effort). Women often give more weight to the individual and seek solutions that help the team and the individual. This results in different managerial styles. When boys are playing a game and someone is hurt, the person leaves the game and perhaps the game continues. When girls play a game and someone is hurt, they are more likely to stop the game (Paley, 1984).

American men give more emphasis to self-reliance, freedom, reason, and power. American women give more emphasis to mutual dependency, caring, feeling, and process. (Note parallels with Eastern-Western differences.)

Understanding and valuing gender differences is an important part of relationship therapy (e.g., marital, premarital) (Gray, 1993; Tannen, 1990). It should also be included in adolescent and teen life-skill courses, such as those taught in public schools. The integrative helper is sensitive to how a gender difference with the client may affect the helping process, and he or she appreciates gender differences in therapeutic goals. Of course, most people possess both male and female attributes, such as those above. It is a matter of degree and balance. For some therapists, such as Jung, cultivating both sets of attributes is an important part of becoming a fully integrated person.

With the rise of feminism as a major force beginning in the 1960s, NAMAP gradually became more aware of female psychological needs and gender biases in our concepts of mental health. For example, many models of psychological health (e.g., Freud) are based on striving for autonomy. But, as discussed above, women often value human connectedness more than autonomy. Traditionally, this might be seen as having a dependent personality disorder. Men's suicides are often related to work or injured pride. Women's suicides are often related to a failed relationship. In her critique of the *DSM* (*Diagnostic and Statistical Manual of Mental Disorders*, mentioned above), Caplan (1995) points out many gender biases concerning what is "normal." For example, the *DSM-IV* includes the diagnostic category "premenstrual dysphonic disorder" (i.e., premenstrual syndrome), through which half a million American women could be classified as mentally ill. Such labeling could then affect job interviews, custody proceedings, and mental competence hearings.

A decade after the women's movement began, men started to realize that inadequate attention was being given to the psychological needs of men. By the mid-1980s, the men's movement had become a force in America (Keen, 1991). And more attention is now given to the therapeutic implications of being male (Kilmartin, 1994; Levant, 1995; Meth & Pasick, 1990). What does it mean to be "masculine" and how does that relate to men's changing roles in the home and the professional world? Issues of concern to men include father-son relationships (their fathers and their sons), fathering and parenting, male bonding, expressing feelings, anger and aggression, recovery from psychological wounds and addictions, pursuit of achievement and money, masculine spirituality, and how all these concerns relate to broader social issues such as child-rearing, education, and social/political problems. And what types of models, such as myths and stories, speak to men about these issues (Bly, 1990)?

Some forms of therapy, such as sensitivity training, are more geared toward cultivating female ways of relating. Other approaches, such as assertiveness training, emphasize more male ways of relating. Group therapy, in which one person talks while others add their perspectives and suggestions, is often more appropriate for women than men. In a group of men, it is often better to let each person tell his story uninterrupted, except for points of clarification. Traditional forms of therapy in which you ask for help, disclose weaknesses, express emotions, cultivate intimacy, and are involved in processes with no clear-cut goals are often uncomfortable for men and they avoid them. Hence, more women than men seek out traditional therapy. New forms of therapy are being developed for men, forms that are more action oriented than verbal. Personal, emotional, and spiritual issues arise in the context of male group activities, ceremonies, bodywork, storytelling, music, and art.

CONJUNCTIVE PSYCHOLOGY

Conjunctive Psychology is an evolving approach that seeks the gradual development of an integrated, multilevel psychology of behavior change and personal growth that draws from all the world's major psychologies (e.g., Mikulas, 1995, 1996b). Let us recognize and take delight in individual differences, gender differences, and other cultural differences. We want to take these differences into account in therapy and also gradually develop a perspective that is superordinate to these differences, including them as special cases.

When I survey NAMAP and/or world psychologies, I find the same phenomena and dynamics described in many different ways. Why choose one model or conceptualization over another? Not being theory driven, models in Conjunctive Psychology can be chosen based on their practical and heuristic values (remember that "heuristic" mean "serves to discover or stimulate investigation"). Which model is the clearest, cleanest, and/or most parsimonious? Which constructs best lend themselves to scientific investigation in the broadest sense? Which theories have the most obvious practical/applied implications? Which models best facilitate seeing diverse interrelationships among constructs in a broad integrated perspective? Of course, what is most useful for one person is not necessarily the most useful for another. Hence, the objectives of this book are to be heuristic, not necessarily provide "the answer."

One example is the construct "behaviors of the mind," discussed in detail later. The heuristic value of this construct, established over several decades of research, clinical applications, teaching, and workshops, includes the following: Use of the construct clarifies some common confusions of Western psychology and philosophy, confusions with widespread, significant, practical implications in therapy, education, and personal/spiritual growth. The construct provides an alternative, logical, powerful approach for behavior therapists, cognitive therapists, and others working with cognitions. The construct facilitates integrating Eastern and Western psychologies. And the different behaviors of the mind can be defined operationally, studied and trained behaviorally, and shown to differ neurophysiologically (Mikulas, 2000).

Another example is the four levels of being, a map that is central to Conjunctive Psychology and the organization of this book. This map is not particularly complex, clever, or unique, but, as argued below, it has strong, established heuristic value.

FOUR LEVELS OF BEING

Conjunctive Psychology recognizes that essentially all people exist at four totally interrelated levels of being: biological, behavioral, personal, and transpersonal. The integrative helper has basic knowledge of all four levels and how they interact.

The biological level refers to the state and predispositions of the body. Therapies might involve working with nutrition, exercise, breathing, environmental pollution, bodywork, or drugs. The behavioral level refers to what the person does, including overt behavior, emotional responses, and thoughts and images. Therapies might involve learning new behaviors and/or decreasing undesired behaviors. The personal level includes the individual's conscious experiential sense of self, will, and personal reality. Therapies might involve discrimination training, the structure of the self or selves, attitudes toward the self or selves, and perceived competency and will. The transpersonal level includes those forces, processes, and domains of being that are superordinate to and prior to the personal, such as those social variables and dynamics of consciousness that construct the personal reality, sense of self, and sense of will of the personal level. Biologically and socially, the transpersonal level includes how the individual is embedded in the family, community, and culture. Intrapsychically, transpersonal forces operate through behaviors of the mind that select, construct, and provide awareness of the contents of the mind that are the essence of the personal level.

Many helpers intervene principally at just one of the levels of being. This includes the psychiatrist who primarily uses drugs, the behavior therapist who focuses on behavior, and the humanistic psychologist who emphasizes self-concept and self-esteem. In some cases, a one-level approach may be appropriate or adequate, but some of the most common and most serious problems arise when the helper intervenes at the wrong level, often due to inadequate knowledge of the other levels and/or a dogmatic attachment to one particular level.

An example of such a case was Tommy, who was irritable and disruptive in his elementary school class. For a few weeks, the teacher tried various rewards and punishments, including making Tommy stay under her desk. When this was unsuccessful, Tommy was sent to the school counselor, who determined that the cause of the problem was desertion by Tommy's dad, who had abandoned the family. When a few months of family-related therapy was unsuccessful, Tommy was sent to a psychiatrist, who diagnosed him as having a hyperactivity problem. The psychiatrist gave Tommy stimulants, which only made things worse. It was later discovered that Tommy's problems were primarily due to an allergy to the fruit his mother added to his morning cereal.

Currently, there are tens of thousands of Westerners seriously involved in some formal type of spiritual practice. An implicit assumption or hope of many of these people is that some spiritual attainment (transpersonal level) will resolve or eliminate basic psychological problems or needs (personal and behavioral levels). However, this seldom happens. So now we have a large number of people looking to psychotherapy as an adjunct to their spiritual practice (Epstein, 1995; Kornfield, 1993). An integrated psychology should be able to accommodate these people. How do changes at the transpersonal level interrelate practically with changes at other levels? What are universal practices of psychospiritual therapy and growth?

Western psychological therapies and integrative models are primarily concerned with the behavioral and personal levels. NAMAP has given inadequate attention to the biological level and little or no attention to the transpersonal level. NAMAP therapists generally have inadequate understanding and training related to a variety of biological variables that often have significant psychological effects, such as general nutrition, food allergies, vitamin and protein deficiencies, imbalances in blood sugar level, breathing style, life force or energy, exercise, somatic therapies and bodywork, biological cycles, electromagnetic radiation, and the weather. In their training, they may never hear any reference to the transpersonal level. In the American Psychological Association, transpersonal psychology is generally seen as a subset or variation of humanistic psychology. But transpersonal psychology and humanistic psychology focus on two very different levels of being—transpersonal and personal.

Almost everyone who studies psychology within NAMAP encounters Maslow's classic hierarchy of needs. Almost always at the top of the hierarchy is "self-actualization," a traditional humanistic and personal level goal. What is almost never mentioned is that Maslow (1968, 1970) came to realize that self-actualization is not the end of development, and he added "self-transcendence" as the new top of the hierarchy, a stage corresponding to the transpersonal level. Maslow was a founder of humanistic psychology and later a founder of transpersonal psychology.

The integrative helper has general knowledge of the key variables at all four levels of being. The helper may emphasize one or more levels because of interest, skills, client population, or helping setting. But the helper remains aware of the other levels and when to refer the client for other assessment and therapy.

Some topics are only adequately understood when considered across all levels. Such topics in this book include health, happiness, relaxation, stress, and disease. Another example is aggression; this single topic alone includes genes, hormones, brain dysfunctions, neurotransmitters, drugs, pollution, electromagnetic radiation, ions, noise, heat, aversive and erotic stimuli, territory, crowding, isolation, deindividualization, frustration, exercise, reduction of reinforcement, interpersonal attacks, modeling, social values, reinforcement of aggression, role of media, psychological illness, personality, level of intellectual functioning, cognitive justifications, image of self, expectancies, attributions, sense of control, and self-control skills, among other variables (Geen, 1990; Renfrew, 1997).

Many of the more important issues for developing an integrative psychology relate to how changes at one level of being influence changes at other levels. For example, changes at the behavioral level (e.g., reducing anxiety, learning new vocational and social skills) often result in changes at the personal level (more positive self-concept, increases in self-esteem and self-efficacy). Conversely, interventions at the personal level (e.g., changes in perceptions, values, and goals) may result in changes at the behavioral level (as via changes in reinforcers and punishers). The key is to understand how and when one would intervene at the different levels. In Conjunctive Psychology there is particular interest in universal somato-psycho-spiritual change processes and practices that cut across all levels.

In Conjunctive Psychology, the four levels are postulated to be interrelated in a hierarchical fashion; they are embedded in each other in a way that corresponds to developmental issues and that suggests the sequencing of treatment components. A simple but important example is that we usually have to deal with biological problems before behavioral problems, behavioral before personal, and personal before transpersonal. There are, of course, many exceptions and qualifications. The integrative helper works on many levels simultaneously, switching emphasis as needed.

Finally, consider some of the heuristic values of the four levels. First, the terms for the levels are easily understood and are used in generally accepted ways. Second, the distinctions between levels correspond to phenomena and constructs that clearly fit particular levels. For example, the "self" is unique and specific to the personal level and is a defining construct for that level. And the contents of consciousness that comprise the personal level are distinct from the field of consciousness that underlies the transpersonal level. Third, once the characteristics, phenomena, and relevant literatures for each level have been specified, this information can be assumed when discussing levels. This simplifies discussions and definitions. For example, in Conjunctive Psychology, behavior modification is simply defined as intervention at the behavioral level. There is no need to include in the definition references to "behavior" or "learning," since these are subsumed under the behavioral level.

The four levels are comprehensive. All psychologies and therapies can be mapped onto the four levels, without necessarily accepting all of the associated assumptions and claims. Thus, many different and disparate approaches are included as pieces of the bigger puzzle. The completed puzzle is more important than whether any one piece is "bigger" or "better" than any other piece. In classes and workshops, the ideas and practices being covered can be placed in the context of the four levels. This helps the student interrelate what is being learned with other bodies of knowledge and experience. In a helping situation, use of the four levels facilitates the helper and client developing a practical conceptualization of the types of problems and appropriate treatments. This helps to catch level errors, tendencies for the helper or client to want to use interventions that are aimed at one level when it would be more effective or appropriate to emphasize interventions at another level.

A particularly heuristic feature of the four levels is the facilitation of seeing interrelationships among various approaches and therapies. Because all four levels are totally interrelated, it is not surprising when changes at one level produce changes at another level. The practical dynamics of these effects are most important. Many of the more surprising, popular, and influential discoveries in NAMAP during the second half of the twentieth century were related to how changes at one level affect another level (e.g., how personality and attitudes affect physical health, the field of psychoneuroimmunology, and the evolving theories by Bandura).

SUMMARY

Currently, one of the most vibrant and significant movements across the helping professions is the development of integrative models of therapy. In North America, the emphasis has been on integrating Western therapies, such as psychoanalysis and behavior modification. Worldwide, the emphasis is more on integrating Eastern and Western psychologies. And this East-West synthesis is now becoming a part of American integration.

In this book, the dominant Western field of psychology is called NAMAP (North American mainstream academic psychology). Although some NAMAP members are offended by pointing out weaknesses or biases in NAMAP, understanding these limitations is helpful when developing more powerful, more applicable, and more integrated approaches to helping people.

Two examples of limitations in mainstream psychology relate to development and religion. Currently, NAMAP does not have comprehensive and practical models of development that include the later stages of development. Also, it does not give adequate attention to the religious/spiritual beliefs and practices of the client.

In the last decade or so, the role of cultural differences has become an important issue in mainstream psychology and in approaches such as Conjunctive Psychology that integrate world psychologies. People from different cultures may differ in many significant ways, such as values, motivation, perceptions, sense of self, and expectations from therapy.

Gender differences are an example of cultural differences. Men and women may differ in their perceptions, values, styles of communicating, ways of expressing emotions, problem solving, and developing relationships.

The organization of the rest of this book centers on the four levels of being: biological, behavioral, personal, and transpersonal. These are described briefly in this chapter and in more detail in later chapters. The optimal helper, the "integrative helper" in Conjunctive Psychology, will have knowledge of the basic dynamics of all four levels and how the levels interact.

AUTHOR'S REFLECTIONS

Many of the practices and theories of the Eastern psychologies have been developed over thousands of years and across some very different cultures, and honed during application. However, for many of these practices there are not yet substantial Western research studies. (Meditation is an exception.) This lack has two interesting implications.

First, a surprising number of Western psychologists refuse to hear or publish anything about these Eastern practices until they have been "proven" by Western-style research. This attitude is both arrogant and inefficient. Of course, it is desirable to apply critical thinking and controlled research to any proposed form of therapy, but Eastern psychologies cannot be optimally researched until they are first adequately understood. More important for the objectives of this book is the heuristic value of considering ideas and practices from Eastern psychologies. Such consideration facilitates opening the mind, challenging assumptions, seeing new relationships, and seeking to learn more. Where all this leads, both for the integration project and for the individual reader, remains to be seen and researched.

The second implication of the lack of Western research on some aspects of Eastern psychologies is the great research opportunities. One can take findings well established by Eastern research and substantiate them with Western research methods. Students and young college professors can thus easily do seminal research. And these are the types of studies that tend to be quoted often in the professional literature and frequently picked up by the popular press. Many people have made their careers by such research.

Gender differences are important in themselves. I would have these become a topic in all premarital counseling and high school courses on relationships. Even when some of the generalizations do not apply, discussion of the topic is very helpful. Understanding the possibility of gender differences is often an important part of marriage/relationship therapy. But the main reason this topic is in this chapter is that I have found it a good way to help some people have a sense of the significance of cultural differences.

Despite the simplicity of the four levels of being, over the last few decades I have found this structure to be a very heuristic conceptualization. For all my courses and most of my workshops, I introduce the four levels. This helps to situate what is being discussed in a broader perspective (perhaps a perspective already known), helps students see interrelationships with other bodies of knowledge, and makes clear that I am not overstating the applicability of what is being emphasized. For example, with a course in behavior modification, I can focus on the behavioral level while recognizing the importance of interventions at other levels. I can make it clear that I do not consider behavior modification the answer to everything and can emphasize how behavior modification interacts with other forms of therapy.

I know many therapists and other helpers who regularly use the four-level model with their clients. They report that it is useful in communicating with the client about various treatment approaches that might be used and how they fit together. This can be particularly important when more than one helper is involved. They also tell me the model is helpful to them and the clients in sequencing interventions (e.g., We will work with your self-esteem, but first we must deal with nutrition and drug issues).

None of this is intended to be philosophically clever or sophisticated, but I know it is practical. And readers can readily alter any of it to make it more useful or heuristic for them.

THOUGHT QUESTIONS

1. How could a comprehensive model of development help a person having a midlife or existential crisis? Describe the specifics for a hypothetical or real case.
2. When and how would you assess a client's religious/spiritual beliefs and practices?
(3.) What examples of Eastern influences do you see in your own life? (If an Easterner, substitute "Western influences.")
(4.) What are some of the differences between Eastern and Western approaches to psychology elucidated in this chapter? What are some you can think of that are not in the text?
(5.) Why are cultural and gender differences important in counseling?
(6.) Considering the gender differences, are women helpers better for women clients and male helpers for male clients?
(7.) In the somato-psycho-spiritual change process, discuss balance.

PART two

THE BIOLOGICAL LEVEL

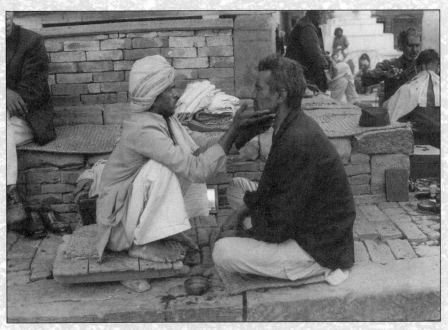

Photo by Benita Mikulas

BIOLOGICAL VARIABLES

The main focus of the biological level is the body, the vehicle through which the other levels take place or manifest themselves. The behavioral level is involved with certain actions of the body. At the personal level, someone's self-concept and self-esteem are often based on the person's perceptions of and thoughts about his or her body, such as how "attractive," healthy, or competent it is. Experientially, a person's sense of self includes the body and/or how a person inhabits and uses the body in various ways. From a transpersonal perspective, the body is part of the role a person is playing in the great play.

EVOLUTION AND LEARNING

Humans are partially a result of biological evolution and are probably still evolving (Murphy, 1992; Wilber, 1995). In the context of Conjunctive Psychology, it is appreciated that evolution can be understood in many ways: intelligent or not; pushed by forces that began in the past and/or pulled toward some goal or source in the future; chance results of scientific laws; meaningful manifestations of the Tao; and/or the creation of God.

An extraordinary development in evolution was the potential to modify the system based on experience. Living beings can learn. Consider the evolution of the synapse, the functional junction between neurons (nerve cells). Instead of a firing neuron automatically triggering the next neurons in line to fire, the synapse allows for more complex interactions. In the synapse, inputs from many neurons are electrochemically added. Both excitatory and inhibitory effects may be involved. And the functioning of the synapse can be altered by learning. As organisms evolutionarily became more complex, with more neurons and more synapses, learning became more important. Rather than adapting by changing biological characteristics (e.g., growing thicker hair), organisms can adapt by changing behavior (e.g., making a coat). A fundamental characteristic of human evolution is that humans were biologically selected for their capability to learn (Dobzhansky, 1972).

Humans are participant-observers in the flow of events of their personal realities. Inventor/futurist Buckminster Fuller defined humans as observers of patterns in the flow of events. This includes a predisposition to notice apparent causal patterns (Testa, 1974). Learning involves changes in the probabilities of behaviors correlated with the observed patterns. (Seeing that Steve enjoys a good joke makes it more likely I will tell him another in the future.) In addition, humans are biologically predisposed or "prepared" for certain types of learning, such as the learning related to language acquisition (Seligman, 1970). Why are certain phobias, such as fear of snakes, spiders, and heights, so common? Seligman (1971) suggests that it is because humans are prepared to acquire such fears. Some apes have an instinctual fear of snakes. Perhaps humans have an instinctual predisposition to acquire such fears. Research support for prepared learning of some fears is complex and mixed (McNally, 1987; Menzies & Clarke, 1995).

Some behaviors, such as basic reflexes and instincts, are largely unlearned, although their form and probability may be altered by learning. Other behaviors, such as playing chess, are learned, although the learning takes place within biological constraints and predispositions. In some situations, it is difficult and/or controversial to separate out learned and unlearned contributions. For example, to what extent are gender differences biologically based? What aspects of "personality" are unlearned? How does the body influence the dynamics and symbols of consciousness?

The integrative helper allows for the possibility of biological components in important individual differences. These biological differences might include reactivity of the nervous system, excessive or defective orienting responses, modal arousal level, relative amounts of inhibition and excitation in the brain, reactivity to stress, ability to experience positive and/or negative affect, and amount and/or efficiency of specific neurotransmitters and neuromodulators.

GENETICS

Genes partially or completely determine some physical characteristics, such as sex and skin color, which strongly influence the type of learning experiences the person has. Consider a boy who is large for his age, as opposed to a smaller boy. The large boy might be more likely to become involved in some sports and thus become more popular. He might be more likely to be called upon or challenged in aggressive situations. And he might be perceived as older than he is and so treated differently.

Is there a genetic component to some psychological disorders such as schizophrenia or depression? Consider schizophrenic parents who have a schizophrenic child. Is this genetic? Perhaps. But it may be that the parents' schizophrenic behavior resulted in the child's learning to act schizophrenic and/or the child's behavior affected the parents' behavior. And what is meant by "schizophrenic?" This is such a vague and general category that two people with very different sets of specific behaviors might be classified as schizophrenic. One set of behaviors might have a genetic component and the other not. And if there is a genetic influence, how does it work?

Research to factor out genetic contributions to psychological problems and traits is very complex, mixed, and beyond the scope of this book (cf. Eaves et al., 1989; Lykken, et al., 1992; Turner et al., 1995); but it is probably safe to conclude that there is evidence for genetic contributions in some cases of schizophrenia (Kety et al., 1994), depression (Moldin et al., 1991), anxiety (Torgersen, 1983), and aggression (Renfrew, 1997). More controversial is whether there is a genetic contribution to some cases of alcoholism and sexual preference.

MALADIES

Damage or dysfunction in part of the body, particularly the brain, may produce psychological effects. For example, schizophrenic-like delusions and hallucinations may be due to Alzheimer's disease (Rubin, 1992), epilepsy (Trimble, 1992), degenerative disorders of the basal ganglia (Beckson & Cummings, 1992), or stroke-caused cortical lesions (Starkstein et al., 1992). Various studies of schizophrenics have found a wide range of brain abnormalities, such as enlarged brain ventricles, dysfunctional corpus callosum, and imbalances in neurotransmitters. Depression is sometimes associated with and perhaps partially caused by Alzheimer's disease (Teri & Wagner, 1992), multiple sclerosis, and Parkinson's disease (Rao et al., 1992).

More generally, brain disorders, such as lesions and tumors, may directly or indirectly, result in numerous symptoms, such as anxiety, irritability, anger, aggression, impatience, restlessness, impulsiveness, worry, sleep disorders, paranoia, mood swings, emotional outbursts, mania, depression, apathy, loss of sense of humor, preoccupation with details, faulty memory, or impaired thinking (e.g., Golden et al., 1983; Prigatano, 1992). For example, a person with a temporal lobe tumor might show signs of anxiety, irritability, paranoia, and outbursts of aggression. If poor, this person might end up in prison; if rich, the person's tumor might be detected.

We are currently in the midst of an explosion of technology for studying brain anatomy and functioning (cf. Bigler et al., 1989; Nadeau & Crosson, 1995). This includes measuring the brain's electrical activity, magnetic fields, blood flow, and metabolic changes. Procedures include the electroencephalogram, computerized tomography, positron-emission tomography, and magnetic-resonance imaging. There is enormous potential here. But we have to be careful not to confuse correlation with causation.

Now what are the implications for the integrative helper who is not a specialist at the biological level? Easiest is when the client has a known brain problem that can be allowed for in assessment and the treatment program (e.g., Horton & Miller, 1985; Webster & Scott, 1988). The helper can learn about the possible effects of the malady and/or consult with a specialist. Second easiest is a brain problem suspected because of a head injury, stroke, infection, disease, cerebrovascular disorder, or use of drugs. Additionally, problems in speech, thought, or vital signs might be noticed.

In other cases, there are some clues that the psychological symptoms have a biological base (Golden et al., 1983):

1. There was a fast onset of the symptoms.
2. The symptoms seem related to other disorders in speech, motor movement, or perception.
3. The symptoms are not correlated with other psychological factors.
4. There is a family history of the symptoms.
5. The onset and change of the symptoms matches known biological patterns better than psychological patterns (e.g., schizophrenic-like symptoms from temporal lobe epilepsy versus many traditional forms of schizophrenia usually develop later in life, lack a family history, and do not deteriorate in the same way).
6. The symptoms are altered by drugs whose effects can differentiate the biological components.

The above examples are all indicators of brain maladies, but the same reasoning applies to other biological disorders. The integrative helper is aware of the types of maladies that are relevant to the problems he or she is working with. For example, enuresis (bedwetting) is sometimes due to a urinary tract infection, which can be detected by a medical exam that includes a urinalysis. Or, when working with sexual dysfunctions, a comprehensive medical exam is critical. A man's inability to have or maintain an erection may be due to anxiety and/or it may have a biological cause such as diabetes, alcoholism, circulation problems, or various medications. A child with learning problems in school might have a vision problem, such as poor development of left/right awareness or difficulty in reproducing in writing what he sees. These types of problems can sometimes be assessed and helped by a vision specialist. A person might seem shy or unfriendly when he has a limitation in seeing or hearing. Thus, in some cases, a helper can be particularly beneficial to a client by arranging for new eyeglasses, a hearing aid, new teeth, or physical therapy.

BIOLOGICAL CYCLES

The functioning of the body involves many complex and interacting biological cycles that have biological and psychological significance (Broughton, 1975; Campbell, 1986; Luce, 1971). Well known are hunger, the sleep-wake cycle, stages of sleep, and the menstrual cycle. Other examples include cyclical changes in body temperature, blood and urine contents, some epileptic seizures, and some cases of mania and/or depression. Possible effects of biological cycles include changes in reaction to drugs, pain tolerance, strength, attention, and cognitive performance.

Disruption of biological cycles can have a host of psychological effects. Best known are the effects when the sleep-wake cycle is disrupted, as when a person works rotating shifts or crosses many time zones when traveling. A person working rotating shifts, and thus sleeping at quite different times, might experience disorientation, fatigue, anxiety, strained family relationships, and greater chance of injury. If the person must stay on such shifts, it is best if the shifts are rotated in clockwise fashion (i.e., days, then evenings, then nights), the shifts last for three weeks or more rather than one week, and days off are provided to catch up on sleep. Jet lag, due to crossing a number of times zones, might result in sleepiness or insomnia, loss of appetite, fatigue, disorientation, confusion, and/or nervousness. Psychological problems, such as depression, might impair sleep, which then makes the person more vulnerable to depression. And some cases of depression might be based on biological cycles or due to disruption of biological cycles.

Circadian rhythms, meaning cycles of about 24 hours, such as the sleep-wake cycle, are often set by light. Jet lag is gradually overcome as the day-night cycle gradually resets the body to the new time zone. Cycles of fewer than 24 hours are called ultradian rhythms and might include hormone levels.

Hormone changes due to daily cycles, menstrual cycles, stress, emotions, and maladies of the nervous system or endocrine system can have a wide range of psychological effects, such as depression, anger, or a sense of loss of control. The field of psychoendocrinology studies how hormones affect behavior (Brush & Levine, 1989). In terms of the life cycle, there are often dramatic hormone changes during adolescence (Buchanan et al., 1992) and menopause (Love, 1997), which may strongly affect perceptions, moods, emotions, and energy. When hormonal effects are suspected, the integrative helper considers for the treatment program such things as exercise, stress management, vitamins and minerals, herbs, and other changes in nutrition and lifestyle (e.g., for menopause, Lark, 1995; Love, 1997).

There also appear to be many seasonal cycles that affect behavior, including seasonal affective disorder (SAD) (Nelson et al., 1990; Rosenthal, 1998). People with SAD experience depression in winter, which alternates with nondepression or mania in summer. These people are predominantly women and the SAD usually begins in early adulthood. There are mixed results suggesting that SAD may be light related. Light-based treatment, effective with some people, includes spending more time outside in the daylight for longer periods, sitting more by windows, and being exposed to light that simulates sunlight. How light influences SAD is unknown, but it may involve effects on hormones (e.g., melatonin, vasopressin, and stress hormones).

Traditional Chinese healing gives great weight to daily and seasonal cycles (cf. Pachuta, 1996). These cycles are held to influence the whole complex of body/mind/emotion/spirit. For example, 3 to 5 A.M. is thought to be a good time for meditation, 5 to 7 A.M. for eliminating judgments and prejudices, and 7 to 11 A.M. for empathy. Particular emotions are more likely to occur during certain seasons: summer—joy, late summer—empathy/sympathy, autumn—grief, winter—fear, and spring—anger. Therapeutically, each emotion is an antidote for another emotion: empathy for fear, joy for grief, anger for sympathy, and grief for anger.

ELECTROMAGNETIC RADIATION

The electromagnetic force (EMF) is one of the four basic forces of nature (the other three being the gravitational force and the strong and weak nuclear forces). A moving electric charge creates an electric field and a magnetic field. An increase or decrease in an electric field creates a magnetic field, and an increase or decrease in a magnetic field creates an electric field. This mutual interaction of electric and magnetic fields is the electromagnetic field. Electromagnetic radiation (EMR) is the propagation of energy through space via electric and magnetic fields. The electromagnetic spectrum includes, in order of increasing wavelength and decreasing frequency, cosmic rays, gamma rays, x-rays, ultraviolet light, visible light, infrared rays, microwaves, radar, and radio waves.

Humans evolved in and are continually bombarded by a wide range of EMR, some of which is reflected and some of which is absorbed by the body. Right now, gamma rays and probably a host of radio and television shows are passing through the reader's body. In addition, humans are generating EMR. Brain waves are a common example; in fact, every atom and molecule generates EMR. We are fields of EMR embedded in other fields of EMR. Thus, it should be expected that EMR has some very basic effects on the body, such as setting and altering biological cycles; influencing the life force; and affecting magnetite, the magnetic crystals in human tissues. Perhaps EMR from one person can influence the behavior of another person, as has been suggested for other living beings (Brown & Chow, 1973).

Increased technology is causing us to be bombarded by more and more EMR from sources such as power lines, radio and TV signals, radar, personal computers and TVs, microwave ovens, cellular phones, alarm clocks, electric blankets, power tools, and electric subway tracks. More than half the gross national product of the earth is based on the EMF. As the body is exposed to more EMR than it evolved to handle, it is experiencing a wide range of biological and psychological effects. There is also the possibility that EMR can be used therapeutically to help heal the body. Becker (1990) provides a summary of both the helpful and healing effects and the harmful and disease-creating effects of EMR on the body.

There are many, but controversial, cases of people developing cancer when living in proximity to sources of EMR, such as power line transformers and substations. Cancer might also be caused by the TV on the other side of the wall the baby sleeps next to, the hairdryer the hairdresser holds near her chest, or the electric blanket one sleeps under (as opposed to using it to heat the bed and then turning it off when one gets into bed). EMR is also suspected of causing birth defects, learning disabilities, alteration in neurochemicals, and allergic responses.

Psychologically, EMR might produce such effects as mood changes, depression, or irritability. These are the types of things the integrative helper needs to allow for. Understanding the client's home and work environment is often an important part of assessment.

Visible light can have a range of psychological effects. For example, in some cases brightening the room may lead to better performance. In other cases, dimming the light may produce better visual acuity and be less fatiguing. Lighting often affects the mood of a setting, which affects the mood of people. Aspects of lighting, such as levels of luminance and color, may produce positive or negative affect in a person, which then influences other behaviors (Baron et al., 1992). And level of illuminance might affect a person's overall arousal level, such as higher levels producing more arousal (Biner, 1991).

WEATHER

Many people are more likely to have positive emotions on a warm and sunny spring day than on a dark and rainy winter night. To what extent this is learned and to what extent it is biological (e.g., SAD) is often hard to determine. But whatever the combination of causes, weather often has a strong psychological influence on people, such as on energy, mood, ability to concentrate, reaction time, and need for sleep (Rosen, 1979). For example, some people are more energetic in cool, dry weather than warm, moist weather; some people feel bad when a change in weather is forthcoming; and some people's sleep is disturbed by low pressure or unstable conditions (Rosen, 1979). In addition, there are individual differences in reactions to conditions such as temperature, humidity, barometric pressure, and ion content.

Some cultural differences are probably partially due to weather differences, although this is too complex to have yet been proven. For example, Europeans in Mediterranean countries are more emotionally volatile and expressive than northern Europeans, perhaps partially due to weather conditions. And what is the effect on a culture's "personality" if it rains a lot (e.g., Ireland) and/or sunny days are rare (e.g., Germany)?

Across time and cultures, one of the most believed weather effects is the phases of the moon (e.g., Lieber, 1978). The word "lunacy" originally referred to a type of intermittent insanity believed to be influenced by the changing phases of the moon (luna). Some police officers, emergency room workers, and psychiatric ward attendants report more activity, agitation, and aggression during a full moon. The prevalence of beliefs about moon effects suggests to some that there must be some truth to it although Western research results generally have not supported influences of the moon on people's behavior (Campbell & Beets, 1978; Rotten & Kelly, 1985).

The best documented and most accepted weather effect on behavior is the relationship between temperature and aggression (Anderson, 1989). Hot temperatures result in more aggression, both within countries and between countries. Hotter regions of the world have more aggression. Hotter years and hotter times of the year and day contribute to more aggression, such as murder, rape, wife beating, assault, riots, and road rage. When talking about anger, we say tempers flare, one gets hot under the collar, or one does a slow burn (Anderson, 1989).

The weather and EMR produce ions in the air, positively and negatively charged atoms and molecules. Nature produces ions by EMR, electrical discharges, and the friction of moving water, sand, dust, snow, or hail. Humans produce ions by polluting the air and by EMR (e.g., power lines). Although the data are mixed, it appears that high concentrations of either positive or negative ions can affect some people's moods and other behaviors (Baron, 1987; Baron et al., 1985; Charry & Hawkinshire, 1981; Soyka, 1977). For ion-sensitive people, negative ions usually produce positive feelings of well-being. Negative ions occur at high altitudes and are generated by moving water, such as waterfalls, rivers, ocean waves, and showers. Air pollution within buildings and cities reduces the amount of negative ions. In some cases, negative ions produce a general increase in arousal and can activate positive or negative behaviors. A person so provoked might feel irritated or act aggressively (Baron, 1987; Baron et al., 1985).

For ion-sensitive people, positive ions generally produce unpleasant negative emotions (anger, irritation, depression, stress, tension, fatigue) and sometimes aggressive behavior. There are many winds around the world, sometimes called "witches' winds" or "devil winds," that are held to have strong impact on some people (Rosen, 1979). This includes the Santa Ana in California, the Chinook in the northwestern United States and Canada, the Foehn in Central Europe, and the Sharav in Israel. A major effect of these winds is a dramatic increase in positive ions, which arrive in the front of the winds. Many things are attributed to these winds, such as increases in negative emotions (above), headaches, nausea, illnesses, accidents, domestic quarrels, murders, suicides, and births. Some people leave the area when the wind arrives. Some doctors won't operate. And the wind has been used as mitigating evidence in court. Although positive ions are a probable component of the effects of these winds, they are confounded with other weather effects (temperature, humidity, and barometric pressure), knowledge that bad weather may be on the way, and a host of psychological beliefs and attributions about the winds. For example, in parts of southern Germany as the Foehn comes in, the air becomes clear, and beautiful views of the Alps that are usually not visible can be seen. But rather than enjoy the beautiful blue sky and spectacular mountain sights, many people become upset and know that bad weather is on the way (respondent conditioning).

POLLUTION

Humans are one of the few complex species that foul their own home and environment. Worldwide, we are polluting our air, water, and food, as with industrial waste. We are poisoning our food sources with preservatives, pesticides, and hormones. In addition to harming our bodies, these pollutants have a range of psychological effects. Sometimes pesticides produce anxiety and depression. Mercury poisoning may be a factor in some cases of autism. Exposure during development to certain pollutants (e.g., organic solvents, dioxins, polychlorinated biphenyls) may cause hyperactivity, attention deficits, reduced IQ, and learning and memory deficiencies.

Worldwide, one of the most prevalent and serious pollutants is lead, particularly for children and fetuses. Lead poisoning often results in lower IQ, mental retardation, hearing problems, high blood pressure, impaired concentration, weakness, depression, irritability, and/or aggression. Lead poisoning might have been responsible for Beethoven's erratic behavior. There is also evidence that lead poisoning could contribute to antisocial and delinquent behavior (Needleman et al., 1996). Lead poisoning may have been a contributing factor to the fall of the Roman Empire (Ackerman, 1990, p. 146). Lead in the air, particularly from gasoline, is a major problem in many cities (e.g., Mexico City, Bangkok). Lead in some candle wicks can also cause toxic amounts of lead in the air. Lead in water comes from lead-based solder and lead-lined cooling tanks. Lead-based paints and lead in the soil are other common ways children get lead poisoning. Additional sources of lead include food cans with seams sealed with lead solder, lead crystal decanters and goblets, some ceramic cookware, some painted dinnerware, plastic bags with lead-based labels used inside out to store food, and some calcium supplements. There are ways to test for and perhaps remove lead in paint, dust, water, and soil. There are also simple tests to discover lead poisoning in children. The Centers for Disease Control and Prevention recommend that children be tested every two years starting at age one, or every year starting at six months if they live in an older home or apartment that has been painted with lead paint. Preventive measures include not letting children chew on things covered with paint; washing bottles, pacifiers, or toys that fall on the floor or ground; washing hands before meals and bedtime; and letting water run for a while before drinking or preparing food with it.

Some people have allergies to certain foods, discussed in the next chapter, or to dust, mold, pollen, or chemicals found in some homes, business offices, and classrooms. Environmental allergies might be due to synthetic fibers, new carpets, cleaning agents, insect sprays, paint, glue, perfume, gasoline, or newspaper print. These allergies may produce a range of biological and behavioral problems, including anxiety, depression, violence, and impaired academic performance. And allergy thresholds can be lowered by stress. The expression "sick building syndrome" refers to a building that seems to be partially responsible for physical and psychological disease, perhaps due to inadequate light, poor air quality, and/or a buildup of many sources of environmental allergens. A Government Accounting Office report suggests that about 20% of all public schools in the United States have air quality problems. Mold is a major problem. Symptoms suggestive of an allergy include pulse increase, breathing problems, rapid behavior change, and dark eye circles or bags under the eyes.

Noise pollution is another common problem, producing hearing deficiencies and stress. For example, one study looked at the effects of chronic aircraft noise on elementary school children, a noise level that affects about 10 million American school children (Evans et al., 1995). The researchers found that chronic noise exposure was correlated with disturbances in the neuroendocrine and cardiovascular systems, deficits in reading skills, impaired memory, poor persistence on challenging tasks, and diminished quality of life. Noise, particularly uncontrollable noise, can also influence aggression in two ways (Geen, 1990): First, it produces stress, which can lead to frustration, irritation, and anger. Second, if the person is already predisposed to be aggressive, noise may activate or intensify the aggressive behavior. Worldwide, noise is increasing at a phenomenal rate. In addition to effects on hearing, we can expect more and more stress-related effects.

DRUGS

A drug is a chemical substance that directly alters biological functions. Drugs can be medicinal, psychoactive, psychotropic (mind altering), and/or recreational. They can be prescribed by a professional and/or part of self-medication.

Medicinal drugs, often prescribed by medical doctors, are primarily for improving the functioning of the body. The integrative helper needs to be aware of psychological side effects of clients' medicines. For example, many medications might produce anxiety, such as thyroid supplements, cold medications, sleeping pills, steroids, and some blood pressure medications.

Psychoactive drugs affect a person's mind—general mood, thoughts, and related behaviors. Included here are arousal-reducing drugs (minor tranquilizers, anti-anxiety drugs), arousal-inducing drugs (stimulants such as amphetamines and caffeine), antidepressant drugs, and antipsychotic drugs. If the integrative helper has clients on psychoactive drugs, then the helper needs to learn about the various drugs, their effects and side effects (cf. Julien, 1997; Leccese, 1991; Poling et al., 1991). This is a difficult literature to keep up with, as new drugs are continually being introduced and side effects are constantly being discovered and disclosed. Psychoactive drugs have many biological and psychological side effects. Anti-anxiety drugs might produce nausea, dizziness, drowsiness, impaired motor performance, slurred speech, decreased concentration, confusion, disorientation, short-term memory loss, and/or depersonalization. Antidepressant drugs might produce blurred vision, constipation, sweating, impotence, insomnia, weight gain or loss, drowsiness, and/or dizziness. The antidepressant Prozac (fluoxetine) may cause agitation, anxiety, insomnia, weight loss, sexual dysfunction, exaggerated feelings of well-being, or hallucinations. Sedative antipsychotic drugs might produce drowsiness, dizziness, and/or fatigue. Antipsychotic drugs that affect the extrapyramidal system might produce tremors, rigidity, drooling, muscle spasms, insomnia, continuous movement of feet, jitteriness, and/or feelings of inner tension. Secondary drugs may be taken to offset some of these side effects, but the secondary drugs usually have their own side effects. For example, anticholinergic drugs may be taken to offset the Parkinson-like side effects of the anti-psychotic drugs. But the anticholinergic might produce nausea, drowsiness, dizziness, blurred vision, constipation, confusion, and/or disorientation.

In rare cases, psychoactive drugs will be part of a person's long-term maintenance program. In other cases, the drug may be an emergency measure to buy time and/or save a life, as with some suicidal clients. And in other cases, the drug is a temporary part of a more comprehensive treatment program, as when it is coupled with behavior modification. In all cases, the integrative helper considers alternatives to the drugs and ways to possibly reduce dosage and/or gradually phase the person off the drugs.

Psychotropic drugs are mind-altering drugs that affect one's perceptions and thoughts about self and reality. (There is not a clear distinction between "psychoactive" and "psychotropic," as both words are often used.) This includes somewhat different states of consciousness (e.g., "stoned" on alcohol or marijuana) to dramatically different states (e.g., "tripping" on psychedelics or hallucinogens). Psychotropic drugs might help a person break set, challenge assumptions, uncover previously unconscious memories or mental dynamics, work through major problems, or penetrate into a new level of being, such as the transpersonal level. Psychotropics thus may be part of a program of personal growth, personal level therapy, consciousness exploration, or spiritual practice (Smith, 2000). From a spiritual point of view, drugs need to be approached with great respect and caution. The Buddha warned against drugs that impair one's awareness. And of the many Western consciousness explorers for whom psychedelic drugs were an important part of their path (e.g., Carlos Castaneda, Richard Alpert/Ram Dass), most came to realize and/or were told by their teachers that there are more effective and less dangerous spiritual aids and practices.

Recreational drugs, including psychotropic drugs, are taken primarily for pleasure. Alcohol is the main example worldwide. Here the integrative helper is concerned with side effects of the drugs, possible biological and/or psychological addiction (Doweiko, 1999), and whether the client is using the drug to escape from or avoid problems that need to be dealt with. What exactly is the source of reinforcement for taking this drug?

Although drugs are often helpful and sometimes necessary, they can bring many problems (Julien, 1997): Few, if any, psychological problems are cured by drugs, and the drugs may interfere with other therapeutic components. Relying on drug treatment may keep the client from learning new behaviors and skills. Drugs usually have widespread and complex effects, including problematic side effects, only some of which we are aware of. There are great individual differences in people's reactions to drugs, and sometimes different effects with different dosages. Some drugs become effective only after weeks of administration, during which time various biological and psychological changes may occur in the client. Also, many people will abuse the drug and/or become addicted to it.

Jacobs (1995) adds many additional concerns: Inadequate attention and importance is given to side effects; clinicians often assume that the mental illness cannot be treated without drugs and that the side effects are less destructive than the mental problem. Although drugs are often simply classified (e.g., antipsychotic), their behavioral and biological effects are not so easily categorized. Some drugs have been classified differently at different times. In the United States, the pharmaceutical companies are almost completely in charge of the studies on which the FDA (Food and Drug Administration) grants approval for new drugs. And the research studies are often poorly designed—for example, they may be too short in duration or lack adequate placebo controls.

Overuse of drugs is a major problem in many places around the world, particularly the United States. By the middle of the 20th century CE (Common Era), the primary and often exclusive approach to biological health in the United States was drugs and surgery. Knowledge about and research into other approaches to health, developed in the United States or brought from other countries, has often been actively blocked by those who profited from the drug and surgery approach. Also, the drug companies were reinforced for developing their own drugs which they could patent and own, rather than discovering curative properties of natural herbs that could not be exclusively owned. In the second half of the century, people in the United States gradually came to discover and utilize "alternative," "complementary," and "holistic" approaches to health instead of, or in addition to, drugs and surgery.

The popularity of various drugs increased in the United States, partially from people's desire for and belief in quick chemical fixes to problems. If one is anxious and tense, it is easier to take a tranquilizer for immediate reinforcement than to gradually learn how to relax the body, quiet the mind, and reduce anxiety. People take drugs to wake up, fall asleep, and become more even tempered, happier, or less depressed. By the end of the century, the pharmaceutical industry was spending billions of dollars yearly advertising nonprescription, over-the-counter drugs, with people in the United States buying tens of billions of dollars' worth of these drugs yearly. More dramatic is that U.S. consumers were spending over 100 billion dollars for drug prescriptions. On top of all of this, alcohol remains the drug which in the United States causes the most bodily harm, psychological suffering, and financial loss.

Examples of all major psychiatric disorders (e.g., schizophrenia, affective disorder) may be primarily caused by drug abuse (e.g., cocaine) (Julien, 1997). Steroids might produce depression. Panic attacks can be triggered by large doses of cocaine, marijuana, or caffeine. Caffeine is the most used drug in the world. It is found in some coffee, tea, cola drinks, cocoa, chocolate candy, and pain medicines. It is often responsible for headaches, racing mind, anxiety, agitation, and insomnia.

TRAPS

Finally, consider three common, significant traps related to biological-level interventions. The first trap, a basic theme of this book, is the level error, the tendency to overemphasize interventions at one level to the exclusion of all others, usually because a person has a particular interest and/or competency at that level. Examples of level errors would be the medical doctor whose total approach and understanding of body health is based on biological interventions, or the psychiatrist who uses drugs to deal with almost all psychological problems. The integrative helper who is a medical doctor is aware that the biological level is totally intertwined with the other levels, so that biological health is influenced by factors from other levels, such as lifestyle, perceptions, attitudes, and beliefs. Research findings related to interactions among levels (e.g., one's attitude toward life can affect heart attacks and cancer) have received considerable publicity. Similarly, an integrative helper psychiatrist may choose to work with people where a biological intervention is an important part of the treatment package, but be aware when the client needs other forms of therapy, perhaps from another helper.

The second trap is the assumption that if one identifies biological correlates of a problem, then therapy should be biological. For example, a person has a set of life experiences that result in depression. Correlated with the depression is a change in brain chemistry, perhaps a change in the balance of specific neurotransmitters. The error would be to assume that treatment of the depression must directly alter these neurotransmitters, as with drugs and/or electroshock therapy. Instead, it may be that intervention at another level, as with cognitive behavior therapy, may treat the depression, which then would cause changes in the neurotransmitters (Seligman, 1975). Research has found changes in the brain's caudate nucleus correlated with obsessive-compulsive disorders. Behavior modification treatment of the psychological problem has resulted in caudate changes back toward normal (Schwartz, et al., 1996).

A third trap is the ease of administration and high profits related to of some biological treatments, such as drugs and electroshock therapy. Instead of spending considerable time and effort helping clients with their psychological problems, therapists often find that it is faster and much more profitable to use a biological treatment that provides immediate, temporary relief from some symptoms. However, this is seldom an effective treatment by itself and may retard or impair the therapy necessary for long-term improvement.

Parallel traps apply to the other levels of being as well. The integrative helper is alert to strong academic, philosophical, social, and economic forces that push or pull therapists into such traps.

SUMMARY

The integrative helper recognizes that there are great biological differences among people that influence their behavior. This includes genetic effects, reactivity of the nervous system, and physical characteristics that have social implications. It is often important to appreciate how such biological factors predispose and limit a person's behaviors, including emotions. These factors usually cannot be altered, but they often must be taken into account.

Maladies of the brain can produce a wide range of psychological problems, such as anxiety, depression, and delusions. These might mistakenly be considered to have a purely psychological origin. Referring a client for biological assessment of brain structure and functioning may eliminate some unnecessary psychological treatment, and related time, money, and anxiety. Knowing the biological limitations then allows the helper to devise a more appropriate form of psychological therapy.

More attention needs to be given to environmental influences on behavior and consciousness, such as in the traditional Chinese health system. The weather can have strong psychological effects on some people, as through ions, temperature, and impact on biological cycles. Pollution is a major problem worldwide, with widespread biological and psychological effects. This includes food and air pollution, noise pollution, and exposure to excessive lead and electromagnetic radiation. The integrative helper realizes that poor air quality or environmental allergens may be the cause of psychological problems.

Although drugs can be a very important part of a treatment program, in the United States drugs are grossly overused for biological and psychological problems. The integrative helper needs to know what role drugs play in the client's life, and possible side effects of the drugs. Nondrug therapies may take longer and require more effort from client and helper, but they may be the better approach in the long run.

Author's Reflections

It seems obvious to me that electromagnetic radiation (EMR) must have a wide range of positive and negative effects on body and mind. Much research is required to determine exactly what these effects are and at what dosages. The politics of knowledge regarding EMR is quite dramatic in the United States. Industries selling products that generate EMR have been very successful at influencing politicians, social legislation, and media reports, to the benefit of the industries. And many academicians' understanding of EMR effects is based on newspaper and television reports. Maybe current doses of EMR from various sources have no adverse effects, as some argue, but maybe they do.

Perception and thinking of the world is usually in terms of matter. People are separate collections of material stuff, such as skin and hair. But matter and energy are interchangeable. People can be thought of in terms of energy, including EMR, rather than matter. People are fields of EMR embedded in many other fields of EMR. From this perspective, it may be easier to see the interconnectedness of things; people are not as separate as is often assumed. This sense of interconnectedness is fundamental to Buddhist and Native-American cosmology and to the mystical/enlightened perspective, discussed later.

Thought Questions

1. What are the interrelationships between evolution and learning?
2. Give an example of a gender difference that has both a genetic and a learned component.
(3.) List some ways in which you see the biological level of being interacting with other levels in your life.
4. When do psychological symptoms suggest biological causes? Give a hypothetical case example.
(5.) Pay close attention to your biological cycles for several days. Determine, based on your observations, when your optimal times are for various activities.
6. What would make you suspect your client has SAD?
7. Summarize the many ways weather can affect emotions.
8. Give a detailed example of how the weather of a particular country could influence the culture of that country.
9. Why are children of poor people more vulnerable to lead poisoning than children of rich people? Give several different reasons.
10. What different things in an office or classroom might impair health?
11. What are the advantages and disadvantages to drugs for psychological treatment?
(12.) At the end of this chapter, the author warns against three traps the integrative helper should be aware of when treating a client. What are these three traps and some of the preventative measures that can be taken in avoiding them?

BIOBEHAVIORAL THERAPY

This chapter is a continuation of the last chapter, with the two sets of topics interacting in complex, conjunctive ways. With many exceptions, here are some differences between the two chapters: Many of the variables discussed in the last chapter cannot be changed and must be worked around (e.g., genetics, maladies, weather), while almost all the variables of this chapter can be changed. Many variables from the previous chapter require changing the environment; most of this chapter's variables involve changes in behavior. Some of the interventions related to topics in the previous chapter require specialized training to be competent and legal (e.g., a medical degree); most of the topics in this chapter can be dealt with to some extent by the integrative helper. And while many of the previous topics do not necessarily apply to the helpers themselves, all of the current topics are very important for integrative helpers, as individuals and as helpers. Finally, this chapter encourages clients to become more aware of their bodies, to realize they can have more control over their physical selves, and to learn skills related to such control.

SENSORY STIMULATION

During prenatal and infancy periods of a person's life, sensory and motor stimulation facilitate development of the body, including the brain; set learning processes into action; and establish early preferences, as for certain types of music and the odor of the mother (e.g., Leon, 1992). Deficits in a sensory system can impair development, create learning disabilities, and be a factor in many psychological problems. Also, some children are overresponsive or underresponsive to some senses and/or have trouble integrating information from different senses. Some of these children can be helped by an occupational therapist or school psychologist who works with the senses.

Throughout history and around the world, sensory stimulation (e.g., scents, sounds, colors) has been used to affect people's thoughts, moods, and states of consciousness (cf. Ackerman, 1990). Such use of the senses is also part of many healing and therapy systems. It is difficult to know to what extent the effects are innate responses to physical properties of the stimulus and to what extent the effects are due to learned associations. If learned, to what extent is the response culturally true and to what extent is it unique to the individual?

Consider, for example, the use of a mantra in meditation, an object of meditation that consists of a sound, word, phrase, or chant. In the yogic sciences and elsewhere, it is held that some mantras have an innate effect on the mind. Transcendental Meditation is based on assigning a person one of a set of mantras assumed to be best for that individual. Other effects of mantras are acquired (respondent conditioning) during initiation procedures, philosophical associations, and personal experience. And some mantras contain already meaningful words, such as "peace" or "Jesus." Consider the psychological effects of the color blue. To what extent are the effects an innate response to EMR of that specific wavelength, and to what extent are the effects learned? What about a Hindu who worships a blue Krishna? And what are the effects of the use of "blue" in English to describe a depressed mood?

One way to seek possible innate effects of sensory stimulation is to look for some type of consensus across systems and cultures. For example, color is an important part of Native American, African, and Asian healing systems; Western environmental sciences; and various maps of domains of consciousness (e.g., the tree of life of the kabalah). Unfortunately, one does not find consensus here, and less as a greater number of systems are considered. The safest generalization is that colors near the red/orange end of the spectrum are usually more associated with arousal and activity, while colors at the blue/green end are usually associated with calm and relaxation. Yellow is often related to intelligence.

Within NAMAP, there is a moderate amount of research on color effects. For example, Valdez and Mehrabian (1994) suggest that more saturated colors elicit more arousal, brighter colors are more pleasant and less arousing (e.g., white vs. black), and darker colors are more likely to elicit components of aggression, anger, or hostility. Their results support reports that a particular pink has a calming and aggression-reducing effect in correctional facilities.

Faber Birren (e.g., 1978), dean of Western color consultants, suggests the following responses to colors.

Red: creative thinking, short-term energy
Green: productivity, long-term energy
Yellow and orange: physical work, positive moods
Blue: relaxation, deep thinking
Purple: tranquilizing
Pink: restful, calming

Extraverts prefer warm colors such as red or orange, while introverts prefer cooler colors such as blue or green.

Ayurveda is the natural healing system of India (Frawley, 1989; Lad, 1985). It includes nutrition, herbal medicine, yoga, massage, meditation, and use of colors. Based on a diagnosis of the client, different colors are prescribed. For example, if the client has excessive pitta (a firelike component), then cooling colors such as blue and green are recommended, while colors such as red should be avoided. The following are some generalizations about color from ayurveda (Frawley, 1989).

White: peace and purity
Blue: peace and detachment
Green: harmony, balance, healing energy
Gold: discrimination

The integrative helper is alert to the possibility of using color to help the client, such as colors of walls, clothes, and flowers, and as part of affirmations and visualizations. To do this, it is necessary to know how specific colors affect the client. For the helper using art therapy, the client's choice of colors may be an important part of diagnosis and treatment.

Smells often have strong psychological effects. A particular smell may elicit a "forgotten" memory, perhaps with associated emotional components. Smells often affect our moods, such as the perfume of a lover or freshly baked bread in a home. Aromatherapy is the use of essential oils from plants to enhance biological, psychological, and spiritual well-being (e.g., Ryman, 1993). The oils may occur in roots, leaves, flowers, seeds, barks, fruits, and resins. Aromatherapy was used by the ancient Egyptians, such as massaging a person with aromatic oils to calm the nerves (Ackerman, 1990). It gradually fell out of favor in the West and then reemerged in the 18th century. Common examples include jasmine to increase alertness, rosemary for memory, and lavender for relaxation. Flower sachets of lavender have long been used to help people fall asleep. The smell of spiced apples is used to reduce stress and avert panic attacks.

Although there is agreement about the effects some smells, particularly lavender, there is no consensus regarding others. There are also great individual differences in people's overall sensitivity to smells as well as their responses to particular scents. Also, some people have allergies or sensitivities to some smells, such as perfumes. Within NAMAP, there is some research on the psychological effects of odors. For example, Baron (e.g., Baron & Bronfen, 1994) has shown that pleasant fragrances may enhance work-related behavior, perhaps by increasing positive affect.

Earlier I mentioned that certain sounds, such as some mantras, are assumed to have basic effects on many levels of being. In the West, from Pythagoras on, there have been reports that certain sounds and music have altered a person's perceptions, moods, and other behaviors (e.g., Giles et al., 1991). Music is often an aid to personal and transpersonal growth (Assagioli, 1965; Bonny & Savery, 1990). And all around the world, drumming has been a way to change moods and states of consciousness, perhaps because the drumming is sometimes related to natural rhythms of the body. For example, drumming is often part of a shamanic journey in which the shaman enters an altered state of consciousness to acquire knowledge and power (Harner, 1980).

In Western therapies, the role of sound/music has been most developed in the field of music therapy (e.g., Hanser, 1987; Ortiz, 1997; Wigram & De Backer, 1999). In some cases, music is used to help the client relax, as in pain management and/or with a dying client. Music might help ground a person who is agitated, manic, or psychotic. In some cases, music is used to help someone acquire motor, social, or conceptual skills. And in other cases, it is used to elicit emotions, memories, and experiences not easily accessible by traditional verbal therapies, as with some autistic children, some developmentally delayed or mentally challenged children, and some geriatric clients. A person who has trouble verbally expressing emotions might be able to express himself musically, such as with a simple instrument. Clients might sing, play an instrument, dance, or otherwise participate in a musical event. Coming together as a musical group might also be therapeutic.

Movement and dance to sounds and music can also be therapeutic, as in dance therapy (Ritter & Low, 1996). Movement or dance can stimulate sensory-motor development, eye-hand coordination, auditory discrimination, and body awareness. They can help increase relaxation, decrease anxiety, and increase energy. And they can be a way to display and work with emotions, and to communicate through metaphor and symbolism.

Touch is discussed in the next section. I could include taste in our discussion. In ayurveda, different tastes are associated with different emotions, and it is suggested that biological and psychological problems are often best treated by way of all five biological senses. But the main point for the integrative helper is to realize that working with the senses can be an important part of therapy, as well as simply making life more enjoyable for the client.

BODYWORK

Bodywork consists of things done to the body by touch (e.g., therapeutic touch, massage) and things done with the body (e.g., somatics, exercise). Continuing the discussion of the senses, the sense of touch is also very important in early development. When an infant is handled and experiences positive and negative tactile sensations, this stimulates the development of the body, such as the stress response. Research at the Touch Research Institute of the University of Miami has shown that tactile/kinesthetic stimulation (body stroking and passive movement of the limbs) of preterm neonates greatly facilitated their development (Field et al., 1986). Expanding on the value of therapeutic touch, the staff at the Touch Research Institute have found that massage reduces anxiety in child and adolescent psychiatric patients (Field et al., 1992), and they are studying the value of touch and massage with a wide range of clinical problems (Field, 1998). Of course, there are individual differences to being touched. Some learning disabled and autistic children respond abnormally to touch. Some people don't like to be touched. And some therapists touch clients in inappropriate ways.

In the West, massage was a primary form of medicine before the advent of the drug therapies. In the East, massage is part of all the major healing systems, such as ayurveda. Massage stimulates the body's natural healing functions. It can reduce stress and anxiety and help clients learn more about their particular stress patterns. There are now many different forms of and approaches to massage (cf. Knaster, 1996).

While much of massage and physical therapy is done to the client, an alternative approach to bodywork is to emphasize the client's becoming more mindful of his or her body and learning to move and hold it differently. This is the field of somatics (cf. Johnson, 1995; Knaster, 1996). As defined by Hanna, somatics is the study and regulation of the body as perceived from within by first-person perception (Johnson, 1995). Somatic therapies (e.g., Rolfing, Feldenkrais, Alexander Technique, Hakomi, Sensory Awareness, Continuum) have been around for more than a century in Europe and North and South America. Somatics is based on the lived experience of body, mind, and spirit with an emphasis on mindfulness of the body, a practical phenomenology. This includes awareness of structure, posture, alignment, movement, resilience, gravity, resistance, and nonverbal communication (e.g., Johnson, 2000). It involves awareness of different bodies, such as the bony body and fluid body. For some clients, it involves recognizing the value of different types of bodies, such as an open body as or a compassionate body. Dance therapy can be approached from a somatics orientation.

A key concept in somatics is "embodiment," how much one is in one's body, as opposed, for example, to how much one is in one's mind. And how does this embodiment vary with time and situation? Kepner (1987, p. 20) suggests that the "degree to which body process is disowned has an important relationship to the severity of pathology and the degree of contact with reality." Some clients need help to become more embodied. The over-intellectual client who is out of touch with his body may have a distorted image of himself and may suffer from psychosomatic problems. Or a person may feel alienated from his or her body, feelings, and emotions, and thus perceive and act inappropriately. On the other hand, some clients need to become less embodied, such as a person whose sense of self is too identified with biological attributes and functions.

Bodywork, including massage and somatics, helps when "something is constricting, restricted, blocked, misused, or out of balance—generally because of excessive muscle tension and habit" (Knaster, 1996, p. xv). These problems can influence blood flow and nerve conductance, restrict movement, and create unnecessary stress and strain. Hence, bodywork can often help one's biological health. But here the focus is on psychological effects.

Bodywork can help with stress, anxiety, depression, vitality, and sexual dysfunction. Sometimes it is the best first step for a client with severe psychological problems; massage or dancing may be the inroad. Gilchrist (1992) suggests a number of ways bodywork may help in recovery from chemical dependency: "the mediation of physical withdrawal symptoms, restoration of systemic functioning following detoxification, interventions in cravings, teaching of new ways to relax, potential access to repressed issues, and, importantly, ability to process those at the somatic level."

A common report of bodyworkers is that clients' memories and emotions are often elicited, including memories with very strong psychological significance, and calling them up can often result in emotional catharsis. This is particularly true of memories related to the body, such as physical or sexual abuse, accidents, injuries, surgery, war, and difficult birth (Knaster, 1996). For example, a boy who is physically abused by a parent may learn to hold his body in a protective and constricted manner and may repress (escape/avoidance conditioning) painful memories of abuse. Later, as an adult in bodywork, as he learns to open and extend his body, repressed memories of abuse flood out.

There are many implications to this type of body memory. For NAMAP memory researchers, it is an unexplored area of how body cues can trigger memories and how memories might, to some extent, be stored outside the brain. For integrative helpers, it suggests a way to access memories that may be difficult to reach through verbal therapies. And for bodyworkers, it emphasizes the importance of being prepared to work with such memories, by being trained in needed psychotherapeutic approaches and/or by working in conjunction with a psychotherapist.

Many therapists (e.g., Gendlin, 1978; Johnson & Grand, 1998; Kepner, 1987) have advocated therapeutic approaches that combine bodywork and psychotherapy, sometimes called body-centered psychotherapy or talk and touch therapy. Several of the somatic therapies are examples (e.g., Hakomi, Rosen Method).

Last is the importance of exercise. When clients live a very sedentary lifestyle, as is common in the United States, this lack of movement may impact them psychologically in ways they are not aware of. As a person's body becomes sluggish, her mind becomes sluggish, and there is often a decrease in energy and perhaps an increase in depression. Often one of the best things a helper can do is get the client to use her body more. A client who begins walking regularly may find she has more energy during the day, thinks more clearly, and overall feels better about her life. In some cases, exercise may cause the release of endorphins (endogenous opioid peptides) that biologically produce positive feelings. Research has shown that exercise or physical fitness training leads to improved mood, self-concept, and work behavior (Folkins & Sime, 1981; Morgan, 1997; Salmon, 2001). It is very important that integrative helpers stay physically fit, for their own well-being, as a good example to their clients, and to appreciate the practical issues involved. A comprehensive fitness program usually includes cardiovascular endurance, muscle strength and endurance, and flexibility.

BREATHING

Of all the possible ways helpers can aid clients, working with breathing is one of the most common and most important. Breath work is a critical part of yoga, Taoism, relaxation training, and many somatic therapies. Breathing and emotions intertwine in complex ways.

Within NAMAP, there is a moderate literature on respiratory psychology, including the biology of breathing, the role of breath in therapy, and the possible role of hyperventilation (breathing too quickly) in many psychological problems (Fried, 1993; Ley, 1999; Timmons & Ley, 1994). For example, breathing retraining, learning slow-paced breathing, is often part of the treatment for panic disorder, especially for clients prone to hyperventilate (Rachman & de Silva, 1996). And breathing training can help some people with asthma, the number one cause of absenteeism in the United States.

One of the most basic and most important distinctions is between chest breathing and diaphragm breathing. In chest breathing, the action of the chest going in and out is what primarily forces air in and out of the lungs. Breathing is usually shallow, shoulders are often hunched over, the abdomen is often sucked in, and the voice may be relatively high and squeaky. Chest breathing is common in emotional and threatening situations; it can lead to hyperventilation or free-floating anxiety. Holding one's stomach in for appearance might lead to chest breathing.

Diaphragm breathing, also called deep breathing and yogic breathing, is based primarily on the rising and falling of the diaphragm, a partition of muscles and sinews between the chest cavity and the stomach cavity. Diaphragm breathing is deeper and slower than chest breathing. When a person breathes in, the abdomen swells, the rib cage expands, and at the end of the inhalation the upper chest expands. Diaphragm breathing is more relaxing than chest breathing and works the lungs more effectively.

It is very important that integrative helpers develop mindfulness of breathing and learn to distinguish chest breathing and diaphragm breathing in themselves and their clients. Seeing a client's breathing, the helper also notes any unevenness and shakiness, pauses and gasps, muscle tension that affects breathing, or abnormal breathing patterns (described below). A client's breathing can be a general indicator of stress/anxiety and the possible need for breath work. Brazier (1995) points out that the breath is a clear indicator of the inner life of the client. The helper notes whether it is shallow or deep, long or short, rough or smooth, and how it changes as the client tells his story. Brazier also suggests that as the client is encouraged to breathe into his pain, some relief may occur or an insight might be triggered.

As a self-control skill, clients learn to be aware of their breathing and how to do diaphragm breathing, both of which are practiced throughout the day. Then, when in an actual, imagined, or simulated situation that produces stress, anxiety, anger, or some other negative emotion, they learn to notice breathing changes (perhaps subtle) and switch to diaphragm breathing to relax and countercondition the negative emotions. Clients and/or helpers can continue further in breath work (cf. Farhi, 1996) by mindfully experiencing breathing and systematically exploring how breathing affects mind and body, uncovering and removing obstacles along the way.

In addition to chest breathing and hyperventilation, Farhi (1996) describes other ways breathing may be impaired, including the following: reverse breathing, in which the abdomen moves in on inhalation and out on exhalation; collapsed breathing, in which the chest is drawn downward, shoulders are hunched protectively, and the stomach is projected forward and down; throat holding with tightening of the vocal diaphragm and muscles of the throat; breath grabbing, when one grasps for the next breath without allowing a natural and beneficial pause; and frozen breathing, in which contracting muscles throughout the body leads to shallow breathing. Improper breathing often produces tension in the upper body, including neck, shoulders, and head, and may lead to headaches.

Breath work is a critical part of yoga (Rama et al., 1979). Hatha yoga includes practices to strengthen the lungs, remove phlegm, and wash out the nose. Pranayama is the yogic science of breath that includes many breathing exercises (Iyengar, 1987; Rama, 1986). Most Hindus and yogis understand prana to be a form of the universal life force, and pranayama as a way to move this energy through the body. Some pranayama exercises alter the depth, duration, or frequency of breathing. Some exercises involve eliminating or expanding the pause between inhalation and exhalation. Other exercises force unilateral nostril breathing.

Pranayama can improve one's breathing and related biological functions. The yogic texts also list many biological diseases that can be helped by breathing exercises. Pranayama may help quiet the mind, which in yoga is important for meditation. In classical yoga (Patanjali) pranayama is the fourth limb of the eight limbs of yoga (Mishra, 1987). The other limbs include physical exercises and postures, meditation, and morality. The eight limbs are a comprehensive, powerful set of somato-psycho-spiritual practices for health and awakening. In Conjunctive Psychology, this awakening is the transformation that results from the experiential discovering of the transpersonal level of being.

The nasal cycle is a biological cycle in which breathing is often predominantly through one nostril and this relative ease and efficiency of breathing alternates between the two nostrils (Rossi, 1986). The period of change ranges from 25 minutes to over 200 minutes. Yogic science has long claimed that one can alter mental and physical states by altering which nostril one is breathing through. For example, breathing through the right nostril is best when one wants to be active, alert, and oriented to the outside world; and it helps active biological processes such as digestion. Left nostril breathing is better for being quiet, passive, and turned inward. Western research is gradually supporting some of these ideas. Researchers now know that relative nostril efficiency is associated with greater activation of the contralateral cerebral hemisphere and with improvements on cognitive tasks related to that hemisphere (Shannahoff-Khalsa, 1993). For example, left nostril breathing tends to activate the right hemisphere more than the left hemisphere, and it improves spatial tasks more than verbal tasks. Parallel results have been found with emotions, where left nostril breathing tends to elicit more negative emotions (Schiff & Rump, 1995).

In Buddhism, cultivating mindfulness of breathing (anapanasati) is one of the most common and most powerful practices (Buddhadasa, 1997; Nyanaponika, 1962; Rosenberg, 1999). This awareness training is traditionally done during formal sitting and walking meditation, and then gradually cultivated throughout the day. Helpers could emphasize situations with biological and/or psychological significance, such as situations that tend to be stressful or elicit anger. Things that can be noted is whether the breath is long or short, fast or slow, obstructed or smooth, and left nostril and/or right. One can watch the breath twirl around the tip of the nose and notice the temperature difference between air coming in and air going out. One can watch the rising and falling of the diaphragm or stomach.

RELAXATION

Essentially everyone can profit from learning to relax more. This might involve relaxing the body and/or quieting the mind. It might involve relaxing one's approach to living, one's vantage point, or one's clinging. Thus, the integrative helper must be proficient in a number of different relaxation procedures (cf. Harvey, 1998; Hewitt, 1982; McGuigan, 1981; Smith, 1985). Three primary relaxation procedures that also package well are breath work (above), muscle relaxation (progressive relaxation) (Bernstein & Borkovec, 1973; Bernstein et al., 2000; Cautela & Groden, 1978; Rosen, 1977), and concentration meditation (Carrington, 1978; Mikulas, 1987). Other procedures include visual imagery, muscle stretching, hypnosis, autogenic training, and biofeedback. To be proficient in a number of these procedures, integrative helpers must have considerable personal experience using the procedures with themselves, they must know how to adapt the procedures to different clients with different needs, and they should be aware of limitations and possible complications related to different procedures.

Choice of relaxation procedure may be based on the client's interest or lifestyle. Perhaps the client is technology oriented, and biofeedback seems more scientific and credible than some other approaches. Or perhaps the client wants or needs to learn to meditate for reasons other than relaxation. Choice of relaxation procedure is often based on where the client experiences stress, tension, or anxiety. If muscle tension is the problem, then a body-oriented approach, such as muscle relaxation, is best. If mental agitation is the primary cause, then a way to quiet the mind, such as meditation, is best.

At the biological level, relaxation reduces the potential harmful effects of stress. And stress is a major cause and/or aggravation of many to most biological diseases. At the behavioral level, relaxation is a self-control skill that can be used to reduce and eliminate unwanted emotions. Also at the behavioral level is the importance of adopting a lifestyle that provides time and encouragement to relax, reflect, re-center, step out of the melodrama of one's life, and perhaps engage in spiritual/religious practices and readings (Easwaran, 1994; Muller, 1999). The lack of calming activities is a major problem in the United States where many people confuse relaxation with engaging in various recreational activities, which, although pleasurable and perhaps therapeutic, are not sufficiently relaxing. Others object to relaxing because it is "wasting time." And many turn to drugs to relax.

NUTRITION

Foods can influence our energy, mood, and state of mind (Ballentine, 1978; Null, 1995; Somer, 1995; Werbach, 1991; Wurtman, 1988). Deficiency of particular nutrients, due to a deficient diet or impaired processing, can yield a wide range of possible biological and psychological problems (Kirschmann & Kirschmann, 1996). Idiosyncratic responses to some foods, such as food allergies or sensitivities, can result in anxiety, irritation, or depression (Orenstein & Bingham, 1987). Understanding biological/psychological health and disease requires knowledge of nutrition, and helpers will often need to add a nutritional component to the treatment program (e.g., Rippere, 1983).

Unfortunately, a glaring deficiency in the training of therapists in NAMAP and the training of medical doctors in the United States is that both groups receive inadequate instruction in nutrition. Until the end of the 19th century, nutritional approaches were a dominant force in Western therapies. Now, in medical practice, they have been largely displaced by drugs. Most therapists learn little to nothing about nutrition. As a result, therapists and medical doctors make many serious errors in assessment and treatment of problems that are nutritionally based.

Thus, a helper might wish to add nutrition as one of her areas of competence. But what about the integrative helpers who are not specialists in nutrition? What should they know? First, one must consider, in one's thinking and assessment, the possibility of nutritional factors, and perhaps refer the client to a nutrition specialist. Second, one must be aware of some of the symptoms of nutritional problems, discussed below, and perhaps collect some relevant data from the client. Third, if a nutritional problem is discovered, the helper may need to help establish a behavioral program related to the client's maintaining desired nutrition. And fourth, helpers need to try to keep up with the fast-changing literature on nutrition for their own personal well-being as well as for maintaining some basic knowledge of the field.

We earthlings currently have the technology and resources to allow everyone on earth to have adequate food and shelter. But for many reasons, mostly political and psychological, this unfortunately is not the case. Malnutrition is a serious problem worldwide, with great biological and psychological implications (Kaplan, 1972; Lozoff, 1989). Between 40% and 60% of the world's children are mildly to moderately undernourished, and in some parts of the world, 3% to 7% of the children are severely malnourished (Lozoff, 1989). Although some effects of malnutrition may change with needed diet, many effects, such as on the central nervous system, are irreversible. Prenatal and postnatal malnutrition, especially during critical periods of growth, can permanently impair biological and mental development. In addition, undernourished infants often receive less social and cognitive stimulation because they "demand and receive less stimulating interactions with caregivers, spend more time in close body contact, and spend less time in exploration of the physical and social environment" (Lozoff, 1989).

Worldwide, the most common nutritional disorder is iron deficiency. About 20% of all adult men, 35% of all adult women, and 40% of all children are anemic; more than half of this anemia is probably due to iron deficiency (Lozoff, 1989). Common results of iron deficiency are tiredness, lack of persistence, short attention span, and irritability. In some cases, iron supplements have improved attention, memory, and motor control. Women during menstruation, pregnancy, and perhaps menopause need extra iron.

Protein-energy malnutrition may result in apathy, inactivity, withdrawal, reduced responsiveness, poor concentration, and irritability. Some children, whom school officials see as cognitively or socially retarded or slow, simply need a good breakfast and lunch with sufficient protein. Some so-called spiritual diets are unbalanced and harmful, and thus not spiritual. People who get a lot of their calories from junk food (empty-calories foods) do so at the expense of more nutritious foods. Alcoholics, who get a lot of calories from alcohol, often have an unbalanced diet and impaired utilization of vitamins and other nutrients. And moods and stress can deplete nutrients—such as stress depleting vitamin C. Thus, with some populations, such as alcoholics (Werbach, 1988) and people with eating disorders (Reiff

& Reiff, 1992), helpers will want to attend to specialized nutritional needs, and perhaps add in some nutritional supplements, such as B vitamins for alcoholics.

Deficiencies in vitamins can be the cause of many psychological problems. For example, deficiencies in the B vitamins might cause tiredness, depression, irritability, nervousness, poor appetite, and/or insomnia. A deficiency of B_{12} might cause depression, mental confusion, and symptoms of paranoia and schizophrenia. B_3 (niacin) has been used successfully to treat some cases of schizophrenia. The field of orthomolecular psychiatry treats mental illness with "adequate" amounts of nutrients, sometimes large doses of vitamins (William & Kalita, 1977). Some clients have diets that are deficient in particular vitamins, but some people are born with or develop a greater need for certain vitamins and/or are deficient in processing certain vitamins. Hence, some people need large doses of some vitamins. Individual differences in needs and responses to various nutrients, coupled with the behavioral vagueness of many psychiatric classifications, makes orthomolecular psychiatry a difficult field, with complex and mixed results. For example, some "schizophrenics" are helped by B vitamins plus zinc and manganese, others by eliminating grain and milk from the diet, and others by adding essential fatty acids.

Some people have strong biological and psychological reactions to specific nutrients or chemical additives in food. In the United States, over 5,000 chemical additives are used in commercial food processing, including artificial coloring and preservatives. MSG (monosodium glutamate), which used to be common in American-Chinese food, can produce headaches, anxiety, and panic. Such responses to particular nutrients are usually called food allergies, although some prefer the expressions "food intolerance" or "food hypersensitivity." Examples would be a person who becomes depressed from eating tomatoes and a person made more aggressive from eating bananas. The most common sources of allergies are wheat and milk/dairy products. Other examples include chocolate, alcohol, tomatoes, citrus fruits, corn syrup, eggs, garlic, peanuts, yeast, shellfish, soy products, and artificial sweeteners. Possible biological reactions include headaches, aches and pains, breathing difficulties, skin problems, diarrhea and/or constipation, digestive problems, fluid retention, food craving, ulcers, and hypoglycemia. Possible psychological effects include anxiety, anger, depression, mood swings, irritability, restlessness, impaired concentration, and behavior problems. For some children diagnosed ADHD (attention deficit hyperactivity disorder), part of the problem is due to allergies to certain foods and food coloring (which may cause cholinergic hyperresponsiveness and beta-adrenergic hyporesponsiveness in the autonomic system) (Marshall, 1989).

A food diary is useful for detecting food allergies and assessing treatments. The client writes down everything he eats and drinks: what, how much, when. In addition, at set times during the day, including one-half hour after most consumptions, he also notes in the diary such things as mood, energy, or state of mind. This is a very important time for the client to be cultivating mindfulness of body and mind, in general and relative to nutrition. That is, the client regularly stops and pays careful attention to such things as breathing, aches, energy, and thoughts. He has to make careful discriminations, such as exactly which emotion he is feeling and how he would rate it as on a 5-point scale. From the food diary, client and helper can assess the overall nutritional quality of the diet and look for patterns suggesting problematic foods. Unfortunately, although the reaction to some foods, such as sugar, may be quite fast, some food allergies do not show up for several hours or a day or more. There are also laboratory tests that may detect the allergy (e.g., blood tests, skin tests, under-tongue tests).

The next step is systematically to subtract and add foods from the client's diet and observe results, as with a food diary and medical tests. For example, in the Simplification Diet Program (Orenstein & Bingham, 1987), one first systematically eliminates suspected foods and observes the reactions for a week. Then one gradually reintroduces potential problem foods back into the diet, one by one at two-day intervals. Sometimes during the first week after a problem food has been removed, the client may suffer withdrawal, and thus feel worse and perhaps crave that food.

Another nutritionally affected factor with psychological significance is blood sugar level, which is controlled through complex homeostatic processes involving the liver and pancreas. When blood sugar level is up, one usually has more energy and more positive moods. Some people become addicted to sugar as a way to keep blood sugar up. When blood sugar (glucose) is down, they may experience weakness, irritability, anxiety, depression, or aggravation of premenstrual symptoms. Blood sugar level can be thrown off balance by large sugar intake, stress, alcoholism, vitamin B_6 deficiency, impaired kidney functioning, or inability to regulate insulin properly. A urine test and a glucose tolerance test can identify some biological problems. Two common diseases with psychological effects are diabetes and hypoglycemia (Lustman et al., 1986; Messer et al., 1990).

In the most common form of diabetes, the pancreas produces inadequate insulin, which results in a low absorption of glucose. With the cells getting inadequate glucose, a person feels tired, weak, and apathetic. A diet low in sugar and fat and high in complex carbohydrates and fiber is adequate treatment for some forms of diabetes and part of the treatment for other forms. Hypoglycemia is an episode of low blood sugar, which may cause hunger, weakness, nervousness, confusion, impaired problem solving and concentration, hallucinations, anxiety, aggression, blurred vision, and slurred speech. It is sometimes mistaken for drunkenness. Hypoglycemia may be due to diabetes, nutritional deficiencies (e.g., amino acids), food allergies, hormone imbalance, reactions to drugs, or one of many biological diseases (e.g., some cancers). In some cases, symptoms regularly occur before breakfast, two to four hours after eating, and after exertion (Messer et al., 1990). For a few people, diet may be a complete or partial treatment: eating four to six high protein, low carbohydrate meals per day; restricting caffeine, nicotine, and alcohol. If diabetes or hypoglycemia is suspected, the client should be sent for medical assessment and perhaps medical treatment.

Nutrition can influence levels of neurotransmitters in the brain, which can have biological and psychological effects (Somer, 1995; Wurtman, 1988). Carbohydrates increase the brain's supply of the amino acid tryptophan, which is a precursor for the neurotransmitter serotonin. Serotonin is thought to contribute to making one more calm, relaxed, and focused. Proteins contain the amino acid tyrosine, which is a precursor to the neurotransmitters dopamine and norepinephrine. These neurotransmitters are probably related to alertness and being energized. Lecithin, as from egg yolks, nuts, and soybeans, is a good source of choline, a precursor to the neurotransmitter acetylcholine, which has been related to memory, sleep, and motor control. Wurtman (1988) suggests eating protein, with or without carbohydrates, for alertness and energy; and eating carbohydrates without protein for a calming, focusing effect. The effects depend, of course, on individual differences and the brain's current needs for particular neurotransmitters. Wurtman also points out that fat slows digestion, diverts blood to the stomach, and thus, slows and dulls mental processes. Clients can learn to observe their own response to particular nutrients and how the effects vary at different times of the day.

People show great individual differences in response to various nutrients, and this often complicates assessment and research. A food diary, mindfulness training, and systematically altering the diet may help assessment. Helpers should also note what medicines and vitamin supplements the client is taking, checking on possible side effects. Other suggestive cues of nutritional involvement would be changes in the client's diet, cravings for certain foods, symptoms that change hour by hour, and symptoms that occur before or after eating and/or at particular times of day. Nutritional effects on biological health might be evident in weight, eyes, or skin color. Check lists and questionnaires, such as for food allergies (Orenstein & Bingham, 1987), may be useful. One or more of many biological tests might be included, such as a urine test, amino acid panel, glucose tolerance test, or allergy testing. A blood test can partially assess vitamins and minerals and liver and kidney functioning. Hair tests identify metals in the body, particularly lead and mercury, but also many other chemical elements, such as zinc, copper, magnesium, calcium, iron, sodium, potassium, aluminum, chromium, and manganese. These elements can affect vitamins, enzymes, nucleic acid, and neurotransmitters. Calcium and magnesium deficiency may result in anxiety, tension, or panic.

AYURVEDA

Ayurveda (pronounced "ah your vay dah") is the healing system of India (Frawley, 1989; Lad, 1985). Here, its psychological aspects are considered, including how they relate to nutrition (e.g., Ballentine, 1978). There are postulated to be three psychosomatic forces called doshas. The first of these, vata (wind), is related to movement and energy. When it is out of balance, the result can be fear, anxiety, excitability, insomnia, and mood shifts. Pitta (fire) is related to focus and contentment. When out of balance, it can cause irritability, anger, aggression, jealousy, and sleep disorders. Kapha (substance) is related to strength and stability. When out of balance, it causes one to be slow, conservative, lethargic, depressed, or an excessive sleeper. Personality types are based on the relative balance of doshas, with different personalities requiring different proportions of the doshas. Doshas influence all psychophysical functions of body and mind. They can be assessed by different pulses and by urine analysis. Based on such assessment and the client's personality type, treatment might involve selected hatha yoga postures (asanas) and nutrition known to affect particular doshas. Taste often reveals the effects of food on doshas. For example, both sweet and sour foods usually lead to an increase in kapha and a slight decrease in vata. Sweet foods result in a decrease in pitta, while sour leads to an increase. A nervous, flighty person should avoid bitter tastes, which lead to an increase in vata. In addition to diet, doshas are also affected by season, climate, and stage of life, which are considered when choosing optimal nutrition.

Ayurveda also includes three properties of mind related to a triad of fundamental forces called gunas: Sattva (essence) is clear, strong, focused, stable, and pure. Raja (movement) is active, agitated, passionate, and creative. Tamas (inertia) is restful, relaxed, heavy, and dull. As with the doshas, each individual has a particular combination of gunas that suggests a specific diet for optimal biological and psychological health. Sattvic foods emphasize fresh foods, including fruit, vegetables, dairy products, nuts, legumes, and grains. Rajastic foods include fermented foods, eggs, cheese, garlic, chilies, white sugar, coffee, and tea. Tamasic foods include fried foods, frozen foods, heavily processed food, overcooked food, red meat, and alcohol.

LIFE FORCE

Throughout history and around the world, many cultures have postulated a basic life force or vital energy, whose presence separates the animate from the inanimate. There are different suggestions about the source of this energy and the forms and pathways it takes through the body. But nutrition and breathing are commonly held to be basic ways the universal energy is transmuted into other forms of life force for the body. Interesting questions are how this life force relates to EMR and to therapeutic touch.

Life force is a central concept in most traditional Asian healing systems and cosmologies. Disease of the body/mind is often related to this energy (inadequate, blocked, or unbalanced) (Kaptchuk, 1983). In Chinese, this energy is called "chi" (or "qi"), and in Japanese "ki." Chi can be influenced by nutrition, herbs, breathing exercises, massage, and acupuncture. Working with chi is also an important part of the Asian movement arts, such as tai chi and aikido.

Chi kung (or "qi gong"), which means "life force mastery," is a complex system of self-healing of body/mind/spirit (Chia, 1983; Jwing-Ming, 1989; Weil, 1990). It works on the quantity, quality, and balance of chi, and on refining, condensing, projecting, and circulating this energy. Practice involves nutrition, breathing, meditation, postures, movement, and lifestyle.

In Indian systems, the life force takes many forms including prana, doshas, gunas, and kundalini. Prana, discussed above, is the life force associated with the breath that feeds all the organs of the body. Disease is often an imbalance in the flow of prana. And pranayama, in parallel with chi kung, is a set of procedures to purify, develop, strengthen, and redirect prana. In ayurveda, the amount of life force energy is influenced by nutrition, breathing, meditation, deep sleep,

CHAPTER 4 BIOBEHAVIORAL THERAPY **59**

wholesome sensory inputs, appropriate sexual activity, and right thinking. Blocked energy is treated with nutrition, herbs, exercise, and change in lifestyle (Frawley, 1989).

Kundalini is a form of the life force that often resides near the base of the spine and travels up and down parallel to the spine (Scott, 1983; White, 1979). As the kundalini rises it passes through and affects a number of different chakras (discussed later), which are centers of interaction of energy, body, mind, and consciousness. Some forms of yoga (e.g., kundalini, siddha, shakti, tantra) include practices specifically geared toward raising the kundalini, and thus speeding up psychospiritual progress. Some people are concerned about casualties from such practices and suggest kundalini should be allowed to rise naturally as a result of other practices, such as meditation and serving others.

Intentional or accidental arousing of the kundalini can produce a wide variety of experiences, such as pain, heat, cold, tickling and tingling, spontaneous body movements, unusual breathing patterns, unusual or extreme emotions, excessive sexual drive, sleep disturbance, arising of repressed memories, distortion of thought, visions, delusions, inner lights and sounds, detachment, disassociation, and change of state of consciousness (Frawley, 1989; Sannella, 1987). Kundalini problems can be treated via ayurveda, pranayama, and chi kung. Ayurvedic treatment might include rest, relaxation, nutrition, herbs, massage, and specific mantras (Frawley, 1989).

Consider a Westerner whose kundalini is unexpectedly aroused, perhaps due to biological change, personal crisis, or spiritual practices. Unfamiliar with kundalini, he is concerned about his unusual body and mind experiences. When he consults a NAMAP therapist, he is diagnosed as psychotic and eventually given antipsychotic drugs. How can the integrative helper distinguish psychotic experiences from kundalini experiences? This question, addressed by Sannella (1987), warrants more attention and research, for kundalini problems should be approached differently from psychosis. Also, it may help the client to know that his symptoms are natural results of kundalini. In some cases, discussed later, we may want to encourage or facilitate the kundalini process.

Sannella suggests a number of differences between the kundalini experience or process and psychosis: In kundalini, one is more objective about oneself and interested in sharing experiences; in psychosis, one is more oblique, secretive, and preoccupied by significant experiences one has trouble communicating about. In kundalini, voices and sounds are perceived as coming from within; in psychosis, they are mistakenly attributed to outer realities. Heat is a common experience in kundalini, and is rare in psychosis. Unusual experiences are more disorganized in psychosis. If one experiences the energy arising in the lower part of the body, going to the top of the head and back down, and stopping at various points of resistance (chakras), it is probably kundalini, although the procession is seldom this orderly. Finally, the kundalini process may last months or years, during which time the person may pass through many different states of consciousness.

In terms of treatment, Sannella suggests that the client accept the process rather than resist it or try to control it, for the process will usually find its own natural pace and balance. If the process is too rapid or violent, it can be moderated by heavier diet, vigorous exercise, and suspending meditation.

In the West, the idea of a basic life force was fairly common until the development of the mechanical man model of Descartes and others. Now in Western scientific models, life force is seldom included. In psychology, something similar to a life force can be found in Freud's concept of "libido" and Reich's idea of "orgone." Some Western therapies do work with energy. For example, polarity therapy works with how energy moves through body-mind-spirit (Stone, 1986). Drawing heavily on ayurveda, but also other disciplines, polarity therapy includes bodywork, nutrition, exercise, and mindfulness. Finally, the idea of life energy or power has been important to Native Americans. And practices for working with energy and power are basic to Native American shamanism and medicine (e.g., Castaneda, 1998, Garrett & Garrett, 1996; Sanchez, 1995).

MINDFULNESS

A central theme of this chapter, this book, and Conjunctive Psychology is the cultivation of mindfulness, which is also critical in yoga and the somatic therapies. So far, "mindfulness" and "awareness" have been used interchangeably. Now it is time to be more specific. "Mindfulness" as a Buddhist concept refers to the bare attention and choiceless awareness of what is being observed. That is, it is just simply noticing, without evaluation, judgment, or elaboration. The mind may judge, and mindfulness is the noticing of the judgment. Mindfulness is not thinking; it is simply being aware of what is happening, including any thinking. Cultivation of mindfulness is the essential Buddhist practice (Nyanaponika, 1962). According to the Buddha, it is the most important thing one can do, for it facilitates everything else one does. Later, mindfulness will be discussed as a "behavior of the mind," at which time its nature and cultivation will be considered in more detail.

The integrative helper is continually looking for opportunities to add cultivation of mindfulness to other treatment components. When learning progressive muscle relaxation, the client should not simply tense and relax muscles. Rather, he should be instructed to observe carefully the feelings of tension and relaxation. When doing stretching exercises, he should pay careful attention to body feelings. Mindfully exploring a pain, rather than resisting it or getting upset about it, often reduces the subjective pain. The helper points out to the client things to be aware of, encourages the client to notice ever more subtle body sensations, and provides practical advice on how to be objectively mindful (e.g., just notice, don't judge). Keeping written records, such as a food diary, often helps a client develop mindfulness. And specific questionnaires related to awareness of the body (e.g., Shields et al., 1989) may be helpful in assessment, research, and development of mindfulness.

We also want to encourage our clients to notice how changes at the biological level of being correlate with changes at other levels. How do breathing and nutrition affect one's moods, thoughts, and state of consciousness? And in the other direction, how do one's thoughts and attitudes affect one's body? How does one's body "solidify" when one's mind solidifies into an opinion or judgment? Mindfully observing the causal interactions between mind and body is a basic part of Buddhist meditation.

Cultivating mindfulness of the body is important for its own sake, but it also develops a more basic and general mindful aspect of the mind. Thus, when one has learned to be more mindful of one's breathing, being mindful of one's emotions and thoughts becomes easier and more likely. An advantage of using the body to cultivate mindfulness is that the body is ever present and often more obvious. For many people, at first it is easier to be mindful of body activities, such as breathing and walking, than more subtle activities, such as dynamics of the mind. Mindfulness of the body can also help one become more grounded and embodied. When one is too caught in concepts, fantasies, ego-centered melodramas, or problematic states of consciousness, re-centering back into mindfulness of the body may be therapeutic.

The integrative helper cultivates mindfulness of her or his body, for personal advantage and also to be more skillful at helping clients in this area. The helper also cultivates mindfulness of the clients' bodies, such as breathing, posture, movement, tension, and facial expressions. This helps in the assessment of biological and psychological problems and in the noticing of biological correlates of emotions, attachments, and therapeutic change.

This overview of the biological level helps us appreciate the complexity of issues facing the helper who wishes to facilitate well-being in the body/mind. It would be difficult for one to be proficient in all the areas touched on, but the integrative helper can understand the basic issues and the questions to ask, and know when to refer the client to a specialist.

SUMMARY

Working with the senses can often be an easy, enjoyable, and effective component of a change program. Specific music or smells can be used to elicit specific moods. Sensory stimulation is part of most of the healing systems of the world (e.g., Chinese, Indian, African, Native American).

A century ago, nutrition, exercise, and massage were important parts of the health system in the United States. Then they were displaced by drugs and surgery. Now they are gradually being rediscovered as important components for health of body and mind.

Working with the body (exercise, massage, somatic therapies) makes the body healthier, which improves psychological health. For example, when the body is sluggish, the mind is often sluggish. Or when the body becomes healthier and more attractive, the person's self-esteem may improve.

Almost everyone can profit by learning to relax more, including relaxing body, mind, lifestyle, and attitude toward life. The integrative helper knows many different ways to relax and how they apply to different clients. Three of the most powerful approaches, which also work well together, are breath work, muscle relaxation, and meditation. Relaxing the body relaxes the mind, and relaxing the mind relaxes the body. Hence, relaxation is critical to the well-being of body and mind—for example, by reducing stress and anxiety.

The idea of a life force is common around the world and is central to Chinese and Indian health systems. Currently, it does not fit some Western medical models of the body. Hence, it is an important challenge, and it will be interesting to see where this leads. The effectiveness of acupuncture is bringing the possibility of life force into Western medicine. And kundalini effects may prove to be important in some psychological problems.

Breath work is one of the most powerful and general practices a helper can do with herself and with clients! It can be used to increase body functioning, relaxation, and utilization of the life force. It is also a wonderful introduction to mindfulness and meditation.

Knowledge of nutrition is one of the most glaring deficiencies in NAMAP and American medicine. Nutrition has strong effects on body and mind. Nutritional effects might be assessed by a food diary and/or referral to a nutrition specialist. Conditions to consider include deficiencies, allergies, diabetes, and hypoglycemia. Ayurveda suggests some heuristic relationships between personality and nutrition.

One of the most powerful and most applicable practices is the cultivation of mindfulness, which is objective, nonevaluative, choiceless awareness. Mindfulness of the body is excellent for bodily health and a good way to cultivate more general mindfulness. Mindfulness should be cultivated during bodywork, relaxation, breath work, and nutrition assessment.

AUTHOR'S REFLECTIONS

The topics of this chapter are important because they are not adequately covered in NAMAP, they include variables that are often significant in a person's biological/ psychological health, and beneficial changes can often be done quickly and easily. Breath work is a good example.

In a two- to three-hour workshop, I can adequately teach people the following: diaphragm versus chest breathing, deep breathing, mindfulness of breathing, deep breathing as a self control skill, and daily time-outs to relax and do breath work. This, in itself, can significantly help many people and be some part of an overall program for others. From this base, I can move into other practices, such as different forms of relaxation, meditation, or pranayama. All of these, of course, would have a pervasive mindfulness component.

For a variety of reasons, in clinical work I often like to do some relaxation training early. First, it shows clients that there are powerful things they can learn that can actually change their lives. For example, if I do muscle relaxation with a client, I will usually get him or her very relaxed, perhaps more relaxed than any time the client can remember. This excites and motivates clients, empowers them, and adds to my credibility as a helper.

Relaxation training may facilitate assessment, as it puts the client more at ease and perhaps thinking more clearly. The relaxation may enhance the therapeutic relationship. And relaxation as a self-control skill can be an important part of other aspects of therapy, such as self-control of anxiety or anger.

After a person experiences what it is like for the body to be relaxed and/or the mind quiet and relaxed, this becomes a frame of reference to use for noticing when he or she is not relaxed. This becomes more important with continued mindful relaxation practice.

Bodywork, including the somatic therapies, is outside of NAMAP. One reason is that the psychological aspects of bodywork have not been clear to psychologists, largely because of the nature of the literature. Fortunately, this has been changing quickly in the last few years through the work of people like Don Hanlon Johnson (e.g., Johnson & Grand, 1998).

Every year more and more studies are published showing the psychological benefits of simple exercise. Often one of the most important interventions is getting the client to use his or her body more. It can be something as easy as daily walks outdoors. This is particularly true in the United States where the people are often very sedentary. Exercise is very logical to many people, including some who might avoid more psychologically oriented treatments (Salmon, 2001).

I think most readers would agree about the importance of nutrition, but keeping up with this fast-changing field is not easy. In this chapter, I give a basic overview of our current knowledge, but more important than the specifics is recognizing when possible nutrition effects need to be assessed by you or another.

Ayurveda is a vast literature with heuristic suggestions about sensory stimulation and nutrition, among many topics. In this book, I introduce a few ideas from ayurveda. Fortunately, in the last few years, authors such as David Frawley and Vasant Lad have brought ayurveda to the West. You can find hundreds of research ideas in this field.

THOUGHT QUESTIONS

(1.) Name the emotional response you personally have with your favorite color and why you think this occurs.

2. A community mental health center has many rooms for different types of therapy. What colors would you paint different rooms and why?

3. Describe the details of a hypothetical case in which dance therapy has psychotherapeutic benefits.

4. What is your current awareness of your body related to posture and gravity?

5. How does your embodiment change with situations? Be specific.

(6.) For the client who is having difficulty accepting embodiment, what are some of the tools the integrative helper can implement to gradually ease the client into an acceptance of his or her own body?

7. Observe your breathing for a day, including the nasal cycle and chest breathing versus diaphragm breathing. What did you learn?

(8.) Describe a few ways breathing can affect a person's well-being, considering all four levels.

9. How would you decide what type of relaxation would be best for a particular client?
10. How and when would you combine bodywork and psychotherapy?
11. How would you add cultivation of mindfulness into the training program of people at an exercise health club?
12. How does a helper's mindfulness of her or his own body facilitate empathy?
13. Why doesn't everyone on Earth have enough to eat?
14. When might you suspect that moods are related to blood sugar level?
15. Discuss your personality in terms of the relative balance of the doshas.
16. For a hypothetical case, describe the types of information you would want a person to collect in a food diary.

BEHAVIORAL LEVEL

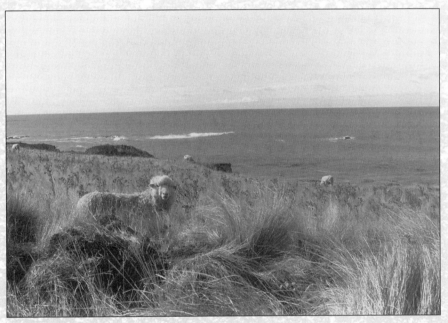

Photo by Benita Mikulas

BEHAVIOR

The focus of the biological level is the body, including the brain. The focus of the behavioral level is how the body behaves, how it responds and acts. The "behavior" of the body includes overt motor behavior, such as walking and talking; covert behaviors, such as thinking and remembering; nervous system activity associated with emotions, such as changes in heart rate; electrochemical activity in the brain; and anything else the body does. In Conjunctive Psychology, "behaviorism" is the study of the behavioral level of being, and a "behaviorist" is a person who emphasizes the behavioral level. Behaviorism was founded by Watson (1913), with B. F. Skinner (1974) as its foremost spokesperson. Note that Skinner's approach to behaviorism is different from Watson's, and many critics of behaviorism misunderstand both approaches. Within and on the edges of NAMAP are many different forms of behaviorism (e.g., methodological, radical, theoretical, teleological, social, cognitive, existential, transpersonal). Some behaviorists restrict their considerations to readily measurable overt behaviors; others include covert behaviors. Skinner assumed that covert behaviors followed the same laws as overt behaviors.

The behavioral level is sandwiched between the biological and personal levels and acts to satisfy their wants and needs. The biological level determines what one is capable of sensing, limits what one can do, predisposes one for certain types of learning, and is totally responsible for some behaviors (e.g., reflexes, allergic reactions). The personal level provides the learned personal reality within which one perceives and behaves. The function of the behavioral level is to satisfy the needs of the biological level (e.g., consummation, pain reduction, homeostasis, sensory stimulation) and to satisfy the wants and goals of the personal level (e.g., conditioned reinforcers such as praise and attention, verification of belief).

Within the constraints and givens of the biological and personal levels, one can explain the dynamics of the behavioral level in terms of the intertwined literatures of learning and motivation (Buck, 1988; Mikulas, 1974; Mook, 1996; Schwartz & Reisberg, 1991; Tarpy, 1997). There are alternative, partial, explanatory systems; but the approach of learning/motivation is the most heuristic, a basic criterion of Conjunctive Psychology. That is, the learning/motivation literatures are the cleanest, most objective, most comprehensive, most integrated, and most researched. NAMAP is very strong in this area, particularly in the psychology of learning; and there are many good texts containing surveys of the NAMAP learning literature (e.g., Anderson, 2000; Barker, 2001; Chance, 1999; Houston, 1991; Schwartz & Robbins, 1995). Therefore, most integrative helpers would profit by taking at least one course in learning or by extensive reading in the area if a course is not possible or practical. Since this literature is very available and known to many readers, considerations here will be on qualifications and elaborations relative to the themes and goals of this book.

A representative NAMAP definition of learning is "the process by which long-lasting changes occur in behavioral potential as a result of experience" (Anderson, 2000). Earlier, a complementary definition described learning as changes in probabilities of behaviors correlated with stimulus patterns. Learning involves changes in behavior potential, what one is capable of doing. What one actually does is also influenced by motivation. Learning is a result of experience with patterns of stimuli, as opposed to other causes of behavior change, such as nutrition or drugs. And this experience may be direct personal experience, or it may occur vicariously, as from watching, imagining, or reading about the behavior and experiences of one-self or another. Aspects of learning may be mediated by symbols, such as words.

OPERANT LEARNING

The best-known form of learning is operant learning in which the probability of a behavior changes as a result of the consequences of the behavior (Ferster & Culbertson, 1982; Pierce & Epling, 1999; Williams, 1973). That is, after a behavior, a person may receive feedback about the consequences of the behavior (Did I turn the wheel far enough? Did I have the right answer on the test? Did they laugh at my joke?) Feedback may produce one or more of the following effects (Mikulas, 1974): It may provide a new learning experience or rehearsal of previous learning (So that's the answer to the test question). It may provide informative cues that guide learning and behavior (I need to turn the wheel more). Feedback may produce changes in motivation, such as changes in goals (I need to study more and work on my joke-telling). It may result in an increase (reinforcement) or decrease (punishment) in the probability of a person's behaving in a similar way in a similar situation. Operant learning stresses this last possible effect of feedback—the influence of reinforcers and punishers.

One of the most powerful and general skills for the integrative helper is the ability to see operant contingencies, how consequences are related to behaviors. Through discrimination learning, you develop the ability to see reinforcement and punishment in most situations involving people, such as the workplace, school, clinic, or home. Those who can see this way are often amazed that others overlook "obvious" powerful influences on behavior.

One approach to developing this seeing has the following three components. First, you learn well the basic operant model and parameters: discriminative stimuli, operant behavior, contingent event (possibly a reinforcer or punisher), and parameters of contingent event (e.g., delay, amount, schedule) (Kazdin, 2001;

Maag, 1999; Martin & Pear, 1999; Miltenberger, 2001; Reese, 1978; Sulzer-Azaroff & Mayer, 1991). You learn about positive and negative reinforcers and punishers, shaping and fading, extinction, and escape and avoidance conditioning. Second, you practice exactly identifying these components relative to behavior in malls, on television, in the workplace, in your family, with pets, and with yourself. Exactly which discriminative stimuli set the occasion for the operant behavior (e.g., sight of beer in the refrigerator, tone of other person's voice)? How can you allow for covert discriminative stimuli, such as thoughts or body sensations? Exactly which behaviors are reinforced and punished in exactly what ways? How do you allow for covert reinforcement and punishment, such as a sense of good feeling from successful accomplishment? With practice, you learn to see operant contingencies all around. Then you add the third training component, altering contingencies. Change undesired contingencies discovered in your own world and establish new contingencies, as discussed in the next chapter.

When one can see operant contingencies in the world, what general things does one notice? Most important, one notices that punishment is used much more than is effective or desirable, and reinforcement is not used enough. One notices many missed opportunities for reinforcing desired behaviors and a surprising amount of reinforcing of undesired behaviors. And one notices many situations where inadequate shaping or fading was the major cause of failure. Fading involves gradually changing the situation, and shaping involves gradually changing the required behavior.

In behavioral assessment with clients, a critical question to ask is, "What is the function of this behavior?" What is the reinforcer for the way the person acts (e.g., social rewards, reduction of anxiety, perpetuation of self-concept)? Skinner was periodically asked how he would solve some social/political problem. He often replied that although he did not know the answer, he knew the questions to ask.

RESPONDENT CONDITIONING

The second major form of learning is respondent conditioning, learning associations between stimuli (Rescorla, 1988; Tarpy, 1997). A song evokes a pleasant memory, a name elicits anger, or a memory brings anxiety. More technically, it is said that in respondent conditioning there is a change in the response to one stimulus (the conditioned stimulus or CS) as a result of its association with another stimulus (the unconditioned stimulus or UCS). As Rescorla (1988) and others have pointed out, knowledge of respondent conditioning is weak and out-of-date in most of NAMAP, mainstream psychology, and psychology in general. There is inadequate knowledge of contemporary findings and theories of respondent conditioning and of many respondent phenomena with clinical import (cf. Davey, 1989, 1992; van den Hout & Merckelbach, 1991). One resulting problem is that NAMAP behavior therapists inadequately understand or work with respondent variables. A second problem is that many behavior therapists prematurely abandoned, in favor of cognitive models, respondent contributions to theories and treatment of fears and phobias.

In Conjunctive Psychology, it is suggested that respondent conditioning involves at least two separate types of learning (Forsyth & Eifert, 1996; Martin & Levey, 1978). One type of learning, CS-UCS contingency learning, concerns what information about changes in the unconditioned stimulus (UCS) is provided by changes in the conditioned stimulus (CS). For example, the onset of the CS may signal the onset of the UCS. This learning, and related behavior, is influenced by many variables, such as unlearned properties of the stimuli, previous learning with similar stimuli, contextual cues, and instructions and expectations. This is the aspect of respondent learning that has been most researched in NAMAP.

The second aspect of respondent conditioning is the simple conditioning of positive or negative affect to the CS. That is, as a result of life experiences, stimuli in a person's world (e.g., people, places, music, memories) come to elicit positive or negative affect, which may be experienced or interpreted in many ways (e.g., like/dislike, love/hate, excitement/fear). Martin and Levey (1978) called this type of learning "evaluative conditioning," and suggested it is more resistant to extinction and less influenced by contingency awareness than is CS-UCS contingency learning. This affective aspect of stimuli has clinical importance. Positive affect is related to addictions, in the broadest sense. Negative affect is related to undesired emotions, such as anxiety, anger, or jealousy. This affect is not easily altered by reason or insight, but is readily changed by behavior modification procedures emphasizing respondent extinction and/or counter conditioning (e.g., exposure therapy, desensitization, and aversive counter conditioning).

Behavioral assessment involves identifying the overt and covert CSs that elicit undesired affect. The client's use of diaries, logs, or checklists might help assessment. For example, a client keeping an anger log might note, soon after each episode of anger, the external situation, thoughts, and feelings that preceded the anger. Simulating situations in the clinic, perhaps accompanied by biological measures, is another assessment procedure. During assessment, the helper uses a problem-solving, concept-formation approach to determining general categories or themes that include the specific CSs. For example, the theme of being anxious about being evaluated may "explain" many of the specific anxiety situations in the client's anxiety log.

TWO-FACTOR THEORY

A classic, heuristic way to understand the interplay of operant and respondent variables is the two-factor theory, or two-process theory (Levis, 1989; Rescorla & Solomon, 1967). According to this view, respondent variables (one factor) often provide the initial motivation and/or consequent reinforcers/punishers for much of operant behavior (the second factor).

For example, Andy, a middle school student, has academic and personal problems that lead him to misbehave in class. The teacher attempts to deal with this by punishment, which respondently conditions anxiety in the boy to the school and teacher. This adds to his anxiety due to academic failings. One day while walking to school, Andy notices his anxiety build (respondent generalization). He stops and goes away from school, which results in his anxiety lessening (operant escape behavior reinforced by the reduction of respondently elicited anxiety). After this, Andy does not even try to go to school (operant avoidance).

Leaving aside considerable complications and qualifications of two-factor theories, there remains a useful scheme for the integrative helper. Prior to most operant behaviors is a motivational state, which may be respondently based (e.g., respondently elicited anxiety or anger). After the operant behavior there may occur a reinforcer or punisher, whose effect may be respondently based. This could be a social reinforcer, such as attention or praise, or a change in the motivational state, such as a reduction in anxiety. Building on the ability to see operant contingencies, discussed above, integrative helpers add in practice seeing respondent and operant interrelationships. Some behaviorists primarily see the operant variables; others focus on the respondent components; some see the rich interplay of the two (e.g., Miller, 1971). A two-factor assessment can facilitate developing a comprehensive, integrated, treatment program and knowing where to intervene first.

In Buddhism, one of the most comprehensive, profound, and least understood models is that of "dependent origination," originally formulated by the Buddha (Buddhadasa, 1992; Nyanatiloka, 1971). According to this view, everything that we experience arises through dependence on something else. In the most popular version, there are 12 links in a circular chain, with each link depending on the previous link. This dependence is stated in various ways. For example, relative to the first four links (ignorance, concept, consciousness, name and form), it is said that through ignorance, concept is conditioned. With concept as a condition, consciousness arises. Because consciousness exists, then name and form arise. Basically, what is described is how biases and lack of wisdom (ignorance) lead to certain body and mind formations (concept), which lead to a particular domain of consciousness and state of mind (consciousness), which lead to a personal sense of mind and body (name and form).

Here emphasis will be on links five through nine, as they relate to two-factor theory. Link five is "six senses" represented by a monkey in a six-window room. The six senses are the five physical senses (seeing, hearing, smelling, tasting, and feeling) plus the mental sense (thinking, remembering, etc.). The monkey, a behavior of the mind, is often drunk or wild and runs from one window (sense) to another, largely out of control. The next link to arise is "contact," illustrated by kissing. Contact occurs when a sense organ, an object of this sense, and related consciousness come together. The eye sees an object and visual consciousness arises. The mind thinks a thought and mental consciousness arises. The next link to arise is "feeling" (arrow in the eye). Here one discerns the immediate affective quality of the sensation, whether it is positive, negative, or neutral. This quality may be innate and/or respondently conditioned, as discussed earlier relative to evaluative conditioning. Some Buddhist mindfulness practices focus on this link of the chain, being aware of this very early sense of feeling.

The next link is "craving" (drinking milk). The affective aspect of feeling leads to motivation, such as to consume or escape. In Buddhist psychology, craving is often the link at which to break the chain. Craving leads to the next link of "grasping" (gathering fruit). Here one tries to hang on to some things and avoid and fight against others. In other words, in the presence of the discriminative stimuli related to feeling and craving, one makes an operant approach or avoidance response (grasping).

Continuing around the chain, grasping leads to things (ideas, experiences, behaviors, and objects) coming into existence for a while (links 10–12 are becoming, birth, death), which then condition the first two links, and so on. For example, a person's intentions, attachments, thoughts, and acts at one instant predispose the body/mind in the next instant to have related experiences, perceptions, thoughts, emotions, and actions. Many of the effects are due to learning. A complete cycle of dependent origination may be very short in time or very long. For most people, a large number of such cycles occur daily. These processes continue to cycle in various forms until a person breaks the chain at one of many possible links. A fundamental goal of Buddhist psychology is getting free from such cycles, as will be discussed later.

MINDFULNESS

Generally, people are not very good observers of their own behavior. So simply asking a client how he behaves in various situations, or why, may not be very helpful. Rather, it may be useful to help the client become a better behavioral observer, and perhaps a recorder of what he observes. This might be done via logs, diaries, checklists, questionnaires, homework assignments, and role playing in the clinic. It is usually best to begin with behaviors easy to observe, such as overt behaviors and strong emotions, and gradually move to more difficult to observe behaviors, such as thinking.

In addition to facilitating assessment, these practices can help the client develop a more generic mindfulness. To encourage this, the integrative helper embeds the assessment practices within more general instructions of mindfulness, as discussed throughout this book. The client learns to objectively and nonevaluatively observe his own behavior and is encouraged to continually extend this mindfulness into broader and subtler domains.

The helper develops mindfulness through practice in observing the behavior of clients and others without judging, evaluating, categorizing, or premature treatment planning. Thinking about what is observed may be necessary or appropriate later; but at first, the helper just observes. This leads to a nonjudgmental and accepting attitude, a basic humanistic goal for a good therapeutic relationship.

Even more powerful is for helpers to practice being mindful of their own behaviors, overt and covert. To do this, they gradually disentangle the "self" from their behavior. The self becomes a witness or observer of behavior. Instead of the experience of I am eating, there is simply the body eating, which is observed by me. (Separating the personal level self from the behavioral level is important to many behaviorists and transpersonalists.)

In addition, when observing your own behavior, simply observe it and try to minimize evaluation, elaboration, or other mental behavior. Later you can think about, evaluate, and perhaps change your behaviors. But for developing mindfulness, at first you should just objectively observe the behavior.

A very important mindfulness component for both client and helper is making friends with yourself, another humanistic goal. That is, you observe and accept yourself, including body and behavior, as you are—for this is "reality." This acceptance does not mean that you will not try to alter reality in various ways, including changing your own behaviors.

BEHAVIORAL-BIOLOGICAL INTERACTIONS

The four levels of being are totally intertwined. Thus, there are many complex interactions between the biological and behavioral levels, a number of which have already been discussed. The behavioral is rooted in the biological; so all behaviors have biological correlates and effects, such as changes in hormones and neurotransmitters. Relatively permanent changes in behavior potential (e.g., learning) require biological changes (e.g., changes in synaptic functioning) (Squire & Kandel, 2000). Also, many variables that strongly affect the body (e.g., nutrition, exercise) come from behaviors.

Some theorists, such as Skinner and anthropologist Gregory Bateson, have pointed out similarities between learning and biological evolution. For example, in evolution, a biological characteristic is generated; and if it is successful, such as improving survival and/or mating possibilities, it is maintained. In operant learning, a behavior is generated; and if it is successful, as in being reinforced, it is maintained. In addition, the distinction between evolutionary changes and learning is often hazy, as when gradual geological changes shape instinctual behavior (Skinner, 1975). All of this suggests more general principles of existence and change that cut across levels of being and include aspects of learning and biological evolution. Taoism emphasizes that all things follow similar and related principles of existence and change (Wong, 1997).

Many varied approaches are investigating how learning interacts with and affects biological processes, such as psychological regulation to maintain homeostasis (Dworkin, 1993). One area of research began with studying how respondent conditioning can suppress or enhance immune responses. Although there was such research in the 1920s and later, the main work began with Ader and associates in the 1970s (Ader & Cohen, 1993). For example, if rats have saccharin (CS) paired with a drug (UCS) which suppresses the immune system, when the rats are later given saccharin and carcinogenic chemicals, they are more likely to develop cancer than rats without such conditioning. In humans, an artificial rose might produce an allergic response, or a cancer patient may become nauseous around stimuli preceding chemotherapy (Ader & Cohen, 1993). Ader named this field of study "psychoneuroimmunology," which includes interactions among behavior, learning, neural and endocrine function, and immune processes (Ader & Cohen, 1993; Ader et al., 1991; Locke & Colligan, 1986; Maier et al., 1994).

The immune system defends the body against infection; it resists toxins and infectious organisms. It was long held to be a biological system that functioned independent of psychological factors. Now we know that there are complex, two-way interactions between the immune system and hormonal systems and the nervous system. On top of this, the immune system can learn, as with the respondent conditioning mentioned above and learning to make quicker responses to specific invaders. As chemicals in food and water can suppress the immune system, so can a host of psychological factors, particularly stress and emotions (O'Leary, 1990; Suinn, 2001). Suppressing the immune system makes a person more vulnerable to many biological diseases. In addition, it can produce fatigue, mental confusion, and/or depression. As the source of stress can come from any level of being, this is a strong example of how the levels are interwoven.

As changes in the behavioral level produce changes in the biological level, so also do changes in the behavioral level produce strong and important changes in the personal and transpersonal levels, as will be discussed later. For example, learning new vocational and interpersonal skills may greatly change a client's self-concept and view of the world. Using knowledge of the behavioral level to facilitate behavioral change is the approach of behavior modification, considered next.

SUMMARY

The dynamics of the behavioral level are best understood in terms of the totally intertwined fields of learning and motivation. The two basic paradigms of learning are operant and respondent conditioning.

Operant conditioning involves learning about the consequences of behavior. The integrative helper learns to ask "What is the function of this behavior?" What is the reinforcement? Do other people reinforce the behavior? Does the behavior result in a reduction in anxiety?"

Respondent conditioning involves learning associations between stimuli. What thoughts and emotions are associated with various people, places, images, and words? Important for the integrative helper is identifying the positive and negative affect elicited by various people, situations, thoughts, and feelings. This includes undesired emotions such as anxiety, anger, and jealousy.

Two-factor theory is a heuristic way of seeing the interrelationships between operant and respondent variables—the two factors. Respondent factors are often a source of motivation (e.g., problems in the workplace elicit anger and frustration). In the presence of specific motivations, the person acts operantly (e.g., stops at a friend's house after work). The operant behavior may be reinforced by respondent factors (e.g., social support reduces anger and frustration).

Cultivating mindfulness of one's own behavior helps clients know themselves better, facilitates assessment, and is a prerequisite for optimal self-control and freedom. Mindfulness of others' behavior is a very powerful skill for integrative helpers.

This involves learning to see operant contingencies, respondently elicited affect, and the interplay of operant and respondent factors.

AUTHOR'S REFLECTIONS

Through experience and practice, you can develop what I call "operant eyes." This is the ability to see operant contingencies in any type of setting, including clinics, half-way houses, classrooms, and businesses. You will be able to go into any such setting and easily see operant variables, such as what behaviors are reinforced and punished, and what discriminative stimuli set the occasion for these behaviors. Based on your observations, you can make practical suggestions. What will be amazing is how others do not see what is now obvious to you.

Developing operant eyes is a very simple skill that is not based on intelligence or book learning. It is basically discrimination learning that can be enhanced by mindfulness. It is learning to see what is already there, but often overlooked. Skinner, of course, had operant eyes. I believe that having operant eyes is one of the most powerful and applicable skills most helpers can acquire.

In the chapter, I outline how to develop operant eyes. In classes, workshops, and clinical training, this learning can be facilitated by continually pointing out examples. Sometimes, the final switch to operant eyes comes on quickly, and the person enthusiastically reports how different the world looks and how obvious many things have become.

When the integrative helper not only has operant eyes, but also respondent eyes and two-factor eyes, then the nature of the behavioral level is largely revealed. The helper can see things that others are trying to assess indirectly.

For many people, including me, there is an incredible elegance and beauty in the processes described by learning. These are basic processes of existence and change, the way the universe moves from one state to another, the functioning of the Tao. Learning cuts across all levels of being. Much of the biological level and the transpersonal level is unlearned. But everything else is based on learning.

Finally, in the chapter I described some correlations between two-factor theory and Buddhist dependent origination. This is the only place anything like these ideas occur. Some variation and expansion of this, perhaps by you, could help integrate Buddhist and Western psychologies.

THOUGHT QUESTIONS

1. Describe the essence of operant learning.
2. How would you assess the role of covert discriminative stimuli and covert reinforcement?
3. Pick an important social issue. If Skinner was a consultant relative to this issue, what questions would he ask?
4. Describe the essence of respondent conditioning.

5. For a hypothetical case of anxiety, describe how you would assess respondent variables and the specifics found.

(6.) Give examples of operant learning and respondent conditioning in your life.

7. Give a hypothetical case illustrating two-factor theory that is different from the ones given in the chapter.

8. Sketch a circular 12-link chain, labeled according to dependent origination. For each link, what pictures and/or words would be most meaningful and evocative to you, regarding the dynamics of that link? How would you use this for contemplation or meditation?

(9.) How does separating the behavior that you dislike in another person, from the real him or her that you love, help in decreasing your resentments and anger toward that person?

(10.) Describe a few ways in which changes at the behavioral level can create changes at the biological level, and vice versa.

BEHAVIOR MODIFICATION

In Conjunctive Psychology, "behavior modification" refers to intervention at the behavioral level. The study of behavior modification includes the theories, practices, research, and training related to such interventions. A representative NAMAP definition is: behavior modification is the application of experimentally established principles of behavior to problems of behavior (Mikulas, 1978a).

As a field of application and research, behavior modification arose in the 1960s, primarily outside of NAMAP. Within NAMAP, experimentalists considered behavior modification too clinical, and clinicians considered it too experimental. In addition, it was challenging the dominant psychoanalytic approach. But logic and effectiveness won out; behavior modification became a strong and accepted part of NAMAP. One of its major contributions to NAMAP was the demand for scientific investigation of the effectiveness of therapies.

Although some use the term in a more restricted sense, since the beginning of the field, "behavior modification" has been the most general term. From this perspective, "behavior therapy" is behavior modification in clinical situations. "Cognitive behavior therapy" is behavior therapy that gives special attention to cognitions. And "applied behavior analysis" refers to operant behavior modification.

There are now many good texts in the field (e.g., Craighead et al., 1994; O'Leary & Wilson, 1987; Spiegler & Guevremont, 1998; Thorpe & Olson, 1997). Hence, this chapter does not survey the literature, but includes discussions of points relative to themes of this book. Consider first some general properties of behavior modification and how they relate to Conjunctive Psychology.

BASIC APPROACH

First, in behavior modification the emphasis is on behaviors, defined and measured as objectively as possible. This, of course, is easier to accomplish with overt behaviors than with covert behaviors. In a behavioral assessment, the question is what does the person do in various situations, rather than what sort of person he or she is (Bellack & Hersen, 1998; Haynes & O'Brien, 2000; Keefe et al., 1978).

And how can these behaviors be objectively defined and interrelated, as with the constructs of learning and motivation? If a person is said to have an "attitude problem," "conduct disorder," or "poor self-concept," what does the person do such that others have labeled him or her this way? Labeling a person, as with psychological classifications, may have some communication value and may be required in some settings. But good behavior therapists and integrative helpers actively try not to label and categorize their clients. Categorizing a person can lead to many potential problems, such as overlooking important behaviors that don't fit the category, assuming that people who are categorized the same have the same behavior problems and/or need to be treated in the same way, and making clients anxious by the labels and perhaps leading them to act in ways they believe people so labeled should act. Rather, it is important to see each client as a unique person with a unique set of behaviors. Similarly, goals need to be specified, as much as possible, in terms of objective behaviors (Mager, 1997). This facilitates treatment planning, confronting practical and ethical issues, and motivating the client.

Second, behavior modifiers try to change behavior directly, rather than produce behavior change indirectly as through insight or attitude change. If one wants a change in a behavior, one should deal directly with that behavior. Historically, many Western therapists and social influence theories have emphasized an indirect approach. The assumption is that general and perhaps widespread behavior change will follow attitude change, insight into the nature of the problem, and/or the uncovering of unconscious motives for the behaviors. These may, in fact, produce behavior change through such things as discrimination learning, change in motivation, and/or changes in values (e.g., what is reinforcing and punishing). This is particularly true when the client has the skills necessary to behave in the desired way but is somehow blocked or unmotivated.

However, in most cases, just changing attitudes, uncovering motives, and facilitating insight is not an effective therapeutic approach by itself. For example, if a client has a strong fear or drug dependency, will understanding how this problem was acquired or being able to interpret the problem in terms of a particular psychoanalytic model cause the problem to disappear or give the person the skills to overcome the problem? Probably not. As London (1969, p. 53) concluded, "After almost 70 years of use, there are still few indications that uncovering motives and expanding self-understanding confer much therapeutic power over most troubling symptoms." Rather, the behavior therapist actively helps the client learn new behaviors and become free from problematic behaviors. For the strong fear the behavior therapist might help the client learn how to relax body and mind and then gradually approach the feared situation, first in imagination and then in real life.

For many decades, social psychologists and others studied how changes in attitudes might produce long-term changes in related behaviors (e.g., behaviors other than those used to measure the attitude). However, as Wicker (1969) concluded, there was "little evidence to support the postulated existence of stable, underlying attitudes within the individual which influence both his verbal expressions and his actions" (p. 75). In addition, although "attitude change" might produce a short-term change in some behaviors, if these behaviors are not independently influenced by behavioral factors such as reinforcement, then the behavior change will not hold (Festinger, 1964; Wicker, 1969). These results had two effects. First has been the attempt of attitude researchers to find better predictors of behavior, incorporating constructs such as past behaviors, social norms, self-monitoring, perceived control, and activation of attitudes and related cognitions (Chaiken & Stangor, 1987). The second effect has been to combine attitude change with behavior modification (e.g., Zimbardo & Ebbesen, 1970). However, most behavior modifiers question the usefulness of postulating an "attitude" and suggest, instead, simply and directly dealing with the behaviors.

Conversely, when one produces behavior change via behavior modification, then insight and attitude change often follow (Cautela, 1993; Mikulas, 1978a). There are many ways this might happen. For example, if a person perceives himself behaving in new, more productive, and more satisfying ways, then his thoughts and perceptions usually change to match, explain, and/or justify these new behaviors. Or when behavior therapy removes problems and obstacles from a client's life, she can often perceive and think more clearly, which creates the possibility for new insights and understandings to arise. This often happens when anxiety is reduced.

In addition, as a result of other aspects of therapy, personal growth, or life experiences, a variety of insights, new perceptions, or changes in values may arise. But for these to be influential in behavior change, they usually have to be encouraged and cultivated through a behavioral action program. New insights or perceptions need to be tried out and honed down through behavioral actions.

Thus, the behavior modifier and the integrative helper both emphasize the need for an active program of behavior change as the most effective way to produce long-term changes in behavior. A common problem in many therapies and personal change projects is that too much time is spent analyzing, reflecting, reading, philosophizing, complaining, blaming, regretting, and so on. There needs to be more action, actually doing something about the problem (e.g., exercise more, join a club, get training for new job, learn self-control skills). This approach of directly dealing with behaviors is similar to aspects of Morita therapy, Buddhist psychology, and the use of commandments and precepts in religious/spiritual traditions.

The third aspect of the basic approach is the emphasis on desired behaviors. Many therapies dwell on the undesirable features of the client, such as problem behaviors or assumed psychodynamic conflicts. This may have some therapeutic value, such as extinction of related emotional responses, but such an approach risks empowering the problem and/or reinforcing undesired behavior. Behavior therapists and integrative helpers put more emphasis on helping clients learn desired behaviors.

A pervasive example of this is behavior modification's emphasis on reinforcement over punishment. There is a common trap here: When things are going well, most change agents (e.g., teachers, parents, managers) do little. Then when a person misbehaves, the change agent springs into action, and punishment is the general response to misbehavior. Thus, most change agents use considerably more punishment than reinforcement. But punishment is usually not an effective change technique. Punishment just temporarily suppresses one behavior without necessarily leading to the desired behavior. Punishment may elicit aggression and conditions in negative emotions to the setting and person where punishment occurred. The punished person often becomes less flexible in behavior and may learn to be more punishing to others. Thus, integrative helpers give more attention to encouraging desired behaviors than to discouraging undesired behaviors.

The fourth aspect of the basic approach is being ahistorical, focusing on the here and now. It seldom matters how the client arrived at where he or she is now psychologically. Rather, what is important is what we are going to do now to help the client move on. If a student has test anxiety, it would be very inefficient and perhaps unethical to spend considerable time trying to determine historically how the student acquired this problem. Rather, the behavior therapist would simply help the student overcome the anxiety. This does not mean one should disregard historical information, but the history is primarily useful to the extent it helps clarify the client's current condition.

The integrative helper recognizes the value of occasionally utilizing a historical context, such as anger-reduction or forgiveness toward a specific historical event, but he or she is cautious of the trap of getting lost in the past. For example, if helpers only seek historical causes, which is the essence of some major therapies, where does that leave the client? Understanding the causes of a problem does not eliminate the problem. And if the causes of the problem are in the past, which can't be changed, this can be immobilizing. Thus, many people unnecessarily feel trapped by a past they can't alter; and many use this as an excuse for staying stuck in their suffering.

The way to get free from the past is to move into the here and now. The integrative helper helps the client become more mindful of and responsible for present experiences and conditions at all levels of being. This emphasis on here-and-now experiences can be found in Gestalt therapy, existential therapy, most major meditation practices, and the transpersonal vantage point. Buddhist and yogic psychologies point out how much time people spend lost in thought, including imaginations of the future and memories of the past. Sometimes something dramatic is required to pull a person into the here and now, such as a beautiful sunset, sexual orgasm, or pain.

Being responsible for one's current condition relates to the fifth aspect of the basic approach, an emphasis on self-control, as much as is possible and appropriate. Instead of doing things to the client (e.g., hypnosis, drugs, psychosurgery), most behavior therapists stress helping clients learn self-control skills that they can use as they see fit (Karoly & Kanfer, 1982). Generally, there is greater and more lasting behavior and attitude change if a client attributes the changes to herself rather than to external agents or special situations (Harvey & Weary, 1981; Winett, 1970). This self-control approach is even more effective when coupled with mindfulness training, as the client learns to observe the behaviors she is working with more objectively and to see chains of behaviors that lead to the problem behavior.

There are many other potential benefits to maximizing self-control. It may encourage the client's cooperation and facilitate generalization and maintenance of therapeutic changes to situations outside the therapy setting. It may make the treatment program more effective and less expensive to the client. And it is usually an effective way to increase positive self-concept and self-esteem, general well-being, freedom, choice, self-efficacy, and internal locus of control in the client.

Some behaviors may take some time to change, and there will be undesirable aspects of the client's world that cannot be altered. Thus, acceptance is an important addition to self-control. The client learns to accept himself as he is, as long as he is actively involved in a change program. And he learns not to unnecessarily upset himself over things he cannot change. The classic serenity prayer applies here: God grant me the serenity to accept things I cannot change; the courage to change the things I can; and the wisdom to know the difference.

Learning Behavior Modification

Problems at the behavioral level are very common—lack of skills that need to be learned and undesirable learned behaviors that need to be changed. In fact, of all client issues dealt with by psychologists, those at the behavioral level are probably the most frequent. Thus, most integrative helpers need to learn about the practice of behavior modification.

Ideally, helpers should take one or more courses in learning and motivation, followed by one or more courses in behavior modification, followed by training and supervision in application. Alternatively, they can read about the field, using the references in this and the previous chapter.

After acquiring some basic knowledge of the field, they should sharpen their practical understanding by trying to apply what they learned. Start simply, perhaps by training a pet or shaping a young child, and then gradually move to more difficult projects. A good way to learn is to do a behavior change project with yourself, such as weight loss, eliminating a fear, or stopping smoking. A number of general self-control books can assist here (e.g., Mikulas, 1983a; Watson & Tharp, 1997), as well as many behavioral books for specific problems, such as anxiety and phobias (Bourne, 1995; Forgione & Bauer, 1980; Goldstein & Stainback, 1987; Peurifoy, 1988), sleep problems (Catalano, 1990; Coates & Thoresen, 1977; Maxmen, 1981; Morin, 1996), obsessions and compulsions (Foa & Wilson, 1991; Steketee & White, 1990), depression (Lewinsohn et al., 1992), weight loss (Jeffrey & Katz, 1977; Stuart, 1983), smoking (Burton, 1986; Danaher & Lichtenstein, 1978), nervous habits (Azrin & Nunn, 1977), and nonassertiveness (Alberti & Emmons, 1975; Jakubowski & Lange, 1978).

Biological Applications

Behavior modification can facilitate biological health in many ways. It can promote those behaviors necessary for the best possible health, such as relaxation, exercise, nutritious eating, and mindfulness of the body. It can reduce psychological factors, such as stress, anxiety, and depression, which are known to cause or worsen many biological diseases, such as heart problems and cancer. In addition, many biological problems often have a psychological component amenable to behavior therapy, such as asthma, pain, and sexual dysfunctions. Relative to medical programs, behavior modification can help increase compliance, reduce fears of procedures, and deal with some of the side effects.

The field of behavioral medicine is the application of behavior modification, in the broadest sense, to biological health and illness (Blanchard, 1992). The field of health psychology includes all of psychology's contributions to biological health (Belar & Deardoff, 1995; Goreczny, 1995; Sarafino, 1998; Taylor, 1999). This book is, to some extent, a text in health psychology.

Discussed later are the ways that behavior modification affects the personal and transpersonal levels. Behavior modification is often the best way to change self-concept and self-esteem, and it clears the way for discovering the transpersonal level. The next chapter examines how behavior modification can be extended to work with fundamental behaviors of the mind.

SUMMARY

Behavior modification is intervention at the behavioral level. Behaviors are changed directly, rather than indirectly through assumed mediators such as attitude change and insight. New desired behaviors are learned and undesired behaviors are changed or replaced, primarily utilizing procedures based on learning and motivation. All behaviors are defined and measured as objectively as possible.

Emphasis is on developing desired behaviors, rather than dwelling on undesired behaviors. The integrative helper learns to emphasize reinforcing desired behaviors and approximations to such behaviors, rather than punishing undesired behaviors.

The overall approach is ahistorical. What are the behavior problems now? Historical factors led to the current condition, but these factors are now gone. Historical information may be useful in understanding the current state, but it is not always necessary.

As much as possible, it is usually desirable to emphasize a self-control approach. Here clients learn skills that they apply themselves, rather than having something done to them. Self-control approaches usually result in more pervasive and longer lasting changes.

AUTHOR'S REFLECTIONS

Perhaps the single most important thing the average person should learn from psychology is the importance of reinforcing approximations to desired behaviors, rather than sitting back when desired behaviors occur and then actively punishing undesired behaviors. The reasons for this are discussed in the chapter.

Opportunities to apply this strategy occur often in most people's daily lives. For example, a manager can expect good work from an employee and comment only when the employee does something wrong. Or the manager can praise desired behaviors, particularly extra effort or changes in a desired direction (e.g., "Thank you for staying the extra half hour; it really helped a lot"). Misbehavior is followed with constructive feedback. With the manager who emphasizes punishment, the employee will not like his job as much, will be absent and late more often, be less cooperative, and have lower self-esteem. With the manager who emphasizes reinforcement, the opposite will generally be true.

Many people are very inaccurate about how much they use reinforcement and punishment. For example, a high school teacher may honestly believe he uses more reinforcement than punishment, but behavioral observation will show he uses punishment more often. Hence, simply telling people about the importance of reinforcement is often not sufficient; they may believe they are already doing it. Rather, there needs to be some type of program that actually results in more reinforcement.

Behavior modification is very effective and often applicable. Thus, some practical knowledge of the field is critical for most integrative helpers. Incorporating behavior modification into their overall treatment approach does not commit helpers to any particular cosmology or theory of people.

When behavior modification first came together as a field, it was very controversial, illegitimate, and not part of NAMAP. Psychologists, social workers, and others developed the field from the outside. Now behavior modification is an accepted, common part of NAMAP, social work, education, and many other disciplines. Currently in the United States, it is often easier to get insurance and other funding for behavior modification than for other forms of therapy, primarily because there is a great deal of research showing the effectiveness of behavior modification, and because behavior modification is often faster and less expensive than some other therapies.

I think the same will be true for some of the topics in this book. Many are not yet well known, many are controversial, and many are challenging the people and ideas in power; but the usefulness and effectiveness of some of these theories and practices will bring them into the mainstream.

I was an observer/participant in the beginning of behavior modification as an influential field. It was fun and exciting. I expect the same will be true for those of you who get involved with some of the new forces that are currently changing psychology.

THOUGHT QUESTIONS

(1.) Describe some similarities between behavior modification and Conjunctive Psychology.

(2.) What "labels" can be applied to you? What emotions do you experience as a result of being so labeled?

3. If a child in a classroom is said to have a "conduct disorder," what might a behavioral assessment reveal?

4. Describe how, in a hypothetical case, behavior modification leads to insight and attitude change. Be specific.

(5.) Describe a scenario in which implementation of behavior modification is not possible without first facilitating insight.

(6.) New insights and perceptions need to be tried out or honed down through behavioral actions. How can this be facilitated with a person who has feelings of inadequency or depression?

(7.) Why is it important to focus on the here and now? What practices could facilitate this?

(8.) How would mindfulness help a client who has problems with aggression?

9. Outline a program to increase your knowledge and skills of behavior modification.

CHAPTER

BEHAVIORS OF THE MIND

7

As mentioned earlier, some behaviorists restrict their study to readily observable overt behaviors, a strong scientific strategy. Internal events, such as thoughts, are defined and studied through overt behaviors, such as verbal behavior about thoughts. On the other hand, since the beginning of the field, some behavior therapists have readily worked with covert behaviors and cognitions (e.g., imagined scenes in desensitization, thought-stopping). Some argue that a "cognitive revolution" took place within NAMAP during the 1970s. From this arose the subspecialty of "cognitive behavior therapy" (e.g., Brewin, 1996; Dobson & Craig, 1996; Foreyt & Rathjen, 1978). Now, most behavior therapists in NAMAP, and probably elsewhere, call themselves cognitive behavior therapists.

Cognitive behavior therapists give particular emphasis to cognitions, such as thoughts, beliefs, and images, and incorporate approaches from various cognitive therapies, such as Beck's cognitive therapy (Beck, 1976) and Ellis' Rational Emotive Behavior Therapy (Ellis & MacLaren, 1998). Cognitive behavior therapists might work with irrational beliefs, thinking style, problem-solving and coping skills, expectancies, or attributions (Spiegler & Guevremont, 1998).

Thoughts and beliefs can be assessed by the client keeping a log of thoughts that occur prior to, during, and after various problem behaviors, such as anxiety or anger. Here the client could be cultivating mindfulness of thoughts. Or the client might verbalize her thoughts while she imagines being in a problematic situation, seeing a videotape of herself or someone else in the situation, or being in a simulation of the situation. Problematical thoughts and beliefs, such as those that are irrational, self-defeating, or particularly negative, can be challenged and/or replaced.

Prior to getting angry, a person might think, "The boss does not like or respect me." A shy person might think, "They don't want to talk to me." During a panic attack, one person thinks, "I will not be able to control myself." And a person with obsessional thoughts might be concerned that "thinking about it increases the chances it will happen."

There is considerable controversy about the effectiveness of therapies that primarily target cognitions and/or assume cognitions to be the primary cause of problem behaviors. For example, many thoughts are quite late in the behavioral chain, such as thoughts that are post hoc explanations and justifications for previous behavior. Such thoughts are not primary, and targeting them would have limited therapeutic usefulness. The integrative helper may assess cognitions as part of a more comprehensive behavioral assessment, and based on the assessment, may or may not work directly with cognitions.

Consider the following somewhat oversimplified cases. When Judy saw people at work talking together, she had the thought, "They are talking about me," which elicited anxiety, which led to other problem behaviors. When Harold was in certain social situations, he became anxious, which led to thoughts explaining his anxiety. Now a simple cognitive approach might work for Judy: Eliminate the irrational thoughts and the resulting anxiety reduces. But for Harold, the cognitive approach would not work; he would still feel anxious, and his mind would find alternative explanations. On the other hand, an anxiety-reduction program would work for Harold, but not Judy. Eliminate Harold's anxiety and there is nothing to explain. But for Judy, the best results possible might be that she still has the irrational thoughts, but they now produce less anxiety. Thus, in our assessment we want to determine exactly how cognitions relate functionally to various behaviors.

Western cognitive theorists basically take one of two approaches to explain cognitions and cognitive change: the conditioning model and the cognitive science model. According to the conditioning model, cognitions are equal to or the result of covert behaviors that follow the basic laws of learning. Thus, specific thoughts and images can be operantly conditioned to change frequency of occurrence, and/or respondently conditioned to change associated affect (Cautela & Kearney, 1986; Upper & Cautela, 1979). These are powerful procedures that are often useful. However, it is the cognitive science model that become dominant in the cognitive therapies and NAMAP in general.

COGNITIVE SCIENCE

Western models of brain and mind have been heavily influenced by the technology of the times. For example, there were the hydraulic models that influenced Descartes, Freud, and the German ethologists. Waterlike forces were stored, mixed, directed, and blocked. Later came the switchboard models that influenced the early American learning theorists. Reflexes, connections, and synaptic changes altered the switches of the brain, such as how a particular stimulus came to elicit a specific response. Currently, NAMAP is obsessed with computer models, although alternatives do exist (e.g., holographic models).

Many NAMAP psychologists are working hard to make the brain seem more like a computer; while many in the field of artificial intelligence are working to make the computer more like a human brain. NAMAP literatures on learning and memory are now dominated by and based on computer concepts, such as coding, storage, and retrieval. Humans have become information processors.

With the computer as the unifying metaphor, the interdisciplinary field of cognitive science came into being; this is an exciting and heuristic blend of psychology, neurophysiology, philosophy, and computer science. Cognitive science, and NAMAP in general, usually make two strong assumptions. The first is that mind and/or consciousness is a product or emergent property of the brain. Thus, for some, if you explain the working of the brain, you automatically "explain" mind and consciousness. The second assumption is that the computer is the best model for understanding the brain. Hence, combining assumptions, the computer metaphor is the way to resolve or avoid basic issues of mind and consciousness.

In Conjunctive Psychology, the wealth of ideas and research findings of cognitive science are valued and incorporated. As these dominate NAMAP, there is no need to discuss them here. However, in Conjunctive Psychology, it is recognized that there are many alternatives to the two basic assumptions, and some of these alternatives may be more heuristic or a better match with the data, at least in some situations. For example, maybe consciousness is not a product of the brain. Many groups around the world think the opposite, that the brain is a product of consciousness.

Maybe the computer is not the best model of the brain. There are many significant differences: Contemporary computer programs are filled with discrete storages, compartments, convergent points, and so on while the functioning of the brain is less discrete and more integrated and holistic. The "information" of the computer is binary; everything reduces to the equivalent of a series of ones and zeros. In cognitive science, this corresponds to the all or none firing of a neuron. But the "information" the brain is processing, through complex, interacting, specific and general, electrochemical activity, is probably not binary. Particularly important is the role of the affect of the information, the positive and negative emotional responses elicited by the information. The affect of what may be perceived influences what is attended to, how it is perceived, the nature and strength of resultant memories, and how it will later be reconstructed for conscious memory. Contemporary computer systems would have difficulties with a component of the information that has such general and varied effects on many stages of information processing.

A "schema" is an important construct in cognitive science and is the workhorse in many theories of cognitive and cognitive-behavior therapy. A schema is a changing cognitive structure that organizes information from experiences and forms a relatively cohesive and persistent structure that influences attention, perception, appraisal, and learning. A schema can have many variables and levels, and there are schemas within schemas. Unfortunately, this is a lot of important psychological functions to load into a nonmeasurable construct. Behaviorally and heuristically speaking, what is added to the therapeutic approach by postulating a schema? In Conjunctive Psychology more attention is given to pulling out, researching, and working with the dynamic forces that are being attributed to schemas.

Conjunctive Psychology is inclusive. It recognizes and honors the approach of cognitive science and incorporates useful perspectives and findings. Integrative helpers also utilize the behavior modification practices of the conditioning model, when applicable, usually in conjunction with other procedures. In addition, integrative helpers have a third approach, focusing on the behaviors of the mind.

Behaviors of the Mind

The construct "behavior of the mind," as described here, is unique to Conjunctive Psychology and has proven to be powerful for integrating Eastern and Western psychologies. "Mind" is meant in a traditional way as the subjective center and agent of mental activity, conscious and unconscious, including perceptions, thoughts, memories, and will. If one is uncomfortable with the term "mind" and/or one assumes that the mind is a product of the brain, then one can substitute "brain" for "mind" in the present discussion.

A very important distinction is between contents of the mind and behaviors of the mind. Contents of the mind include the various objects that arise in a person's consciousness, such as perceptual experiences, verbal and visual thoughts, reconstructed memories, attributions and beliefs, and cognitive aspects of emotions and attitudes. Behaviors of the mind are those processes of the mind that select and construct the contents and that focus on and provide awareness of the contents. Behaviors of the mind occur prior to, during, and in response to any particular contents. Western psychologists and philosophers often confuse and confound contents of the mind with behaviors of the mind.

Three behaviors of the mind discussed below are concentration, mindfulness, and clinging. Concentration refers to the focus of the mind. Mindfulness involves the awareness of the mind, including properties of breadth and clarity. Clinging refers to the tendency of the mind to grasp for and cling to certain contents of the mind and personal frames of references.

The "behavior" part of "behaviors of the mind" recognizes that this is how the mind behaves, what it does, how it responds. These behaviors are influenced by the same general principles of behavior and behavior change that affect all behaviors (e.g., learning and motivation). Hence, behaviors of the mind have learned and unlearned components, can be operantly and respondently conditioned, and can be shaped and tied to specific stimuli. Principles of discrimination, generalization, and transfer are applicable. This is a new and important domain for behavior modification.

There are at least five ways by which current research is establishing the validity of these behaviors of the mind. First is to provide subjects with particular instructions and/or training that produce changes in the behavior, such as how to focus and concentrate one's attention. Second is to solicit the subjects' self-reports of a behavior, particularly when they have had training in the behavior. For example, when hearing a click, subjects might report on a 10-point scale how concentrated their minds are. Third is to study biological correlates (e.g., EEG, event-related potentials) that identify and discriminate between different behaviors of the mind (Dunn et al., 1999; Mikulas, 2000). Fourth is to study the effect of behaviors of the mind on other behaviors. For example, training in concentration might be a component in treatment of insomnia or improving study skills. Objective measures might be time to fall asleep or improvement in grade point average. Fifth, and perhaps the most convincing for most people, is to study these behaviors within themselves, perhaps in the context of mental training, personal growth, and/or meditation.

Behaviors of the mind are, for practical purposes, always present; they can potentially be identified and worked with in any situation. This is why they have such broad implications and applications in many areas, including health, education, counseling, and sports (Mikulas, 2000). Meditation is one situation in which concentration and mindfulness are readily cultivated and have been extensively studied.

MEDITATION

Meditation is a central component in all major Eastern psychologies, and there is now a sizable Western scientific literature on it (Kwee, 1990; Murphy & Donovan, 1997; Shapiro & Walsh, 1984; West, 1987). The practice of meditation can be divided into four components: form, object, attitude, and behavior of the mind.

Form refers to what one does with the body during meditation. In Buddhism, there are four basic forms: sitting, lying, standing, and walking. The integrative helper chooses a form that best suits the client, such as running, swimming, fishing, craft work, or listening to music.

The object of meditation refers to the primary stimulus of one's attention during meditation. This might be one's breathing, an external visual or auditory stimulus, a sound or phrase said to oneself, or an imagined being or scene. The breath is the most used object worldwide, and perhaps the best object for most people. Breathing is very natural and always available as an object. It does not require any philosophical or religious association, and thus is compatible with many. And many important lessons about life and existence can be discovered in breathing. The advantages of mindfully working with breathing were discussed earlier.

Whether a particular practice of meditation is primarily therapeutic, religious, occult, or something else usually depends on the object of meditation. Christian meditation might focus on Jesus and events of his life. A Tibetan Buddhist might meditate on a pictorial representation of the enlightened mind (a type or aspect of a mandala). Therapeutically, a client might be encouraged to meditate on a person or event with clinical significance, and perhaps couple this with a loving-kindness meditation (Salzberg, 1997).

The attitude of meditation is the mental set in which one approaches meditation (Nairn, 1999; Suzuki, 1970). This includes moods, associations, expectations, and intentions. Optimal practice involves persistent dedication, a welcoming openness to experience, a readiness to let go, letting be rather than trying to accomplish something, making friends with oneself, being in the here and now, and perceiving clearly. The attitude of meditation can be heavily influenced by the context in which meditation occurs, such as the context of formal therapy and/or an established psychospiritual tradition. Thus a client's attitude toward meditation might be influenced by his relationship to his therapist, his spiritual teacher, and/or the teachings of a particular discipline.

The fourth component of meditation refers to which behaviors of the mind are being cultivated. If you survey all the major meditation traditions of the world, you find that all of them stress the development of concentration and/or mindfulness (Goleman, 1988; Ornstein, 1986). Thus, meditation can be partially defined as the systematic cultivation of concentration and/or mindfulness. This is quite different from how the word "meditation" is often used in the United States, where it might refer to thinking, day-dreaming, or guided imagery.

Concentration and mindfulness are often best worked with first in a simple situation, such as a sitting breath meditation; but this is not necessary and may not be optimal for a particular client. The integrative helper is always looking for ways to develop concentration and mindfulness in the context of other behaviors. For example, a client might develop his concentration in the context of listening during communication training, focusing on his body during progressive muscle relaxation, or playing a video game. And this book is filled with suggestions for cultivating mindfulness, a central theme across all levels of being.

CONCENTRATION

Concentration is the learned control of the focus of one's attention. It is the behavior of keeping one's awareness, with varying degrees of one-pointedness, on a particular set of contents of the mind. William James (1890, p. 424) suggested that concentration "is the very root of judgement, character, and will" and an "education which should improve this faculty would be the education par excellence."

Poor concentration manifests in many ways. A student may have trouble studying because his mind keeps wandering away from the text. A music lover can't fully enjoy a piece of music because his mind keeps going away from the music, as to thoughts about the music. An insomniac may have trouble getting to sleep because she lies in bed thinking about the next day's problems, unable to put these out of her mind. Many depressive, worrying, and angry clients can't control the arising of negative thoughts and where they automatically lead. Many people are poor listeners, particularly of important and/or emotional topics, because when others are talking, rather than really listening well, they are reacting, evaluating, and planning what to say. In Eastern psychologies, the mind is often described as a wild or drunken monkey. In one metaphor, the monkey lives in a room with six windows corresponding to the six senses, the five physical senses and the mental sense of thoughts, memories, and fantasies. The drunken monkey runs out of control from window to window. Developing concentration involves taming the monkey, not killing it. One learns how to quiet the monkey and keep her or him at the window of choice. The monkey is a good slave, but a bad master.

Concentration is readily developed via meditation (Ellwood, 1983; Solé-Leris, 1986). Consider a sitting meditator watching her breath. Whenever her mind runs off to another object of consciousness, the meditator gently but firmly brings the attention back to the breath. She does not try to forcibly hold her attention on the breath or try to keep other objects out of consciousness. She simply continues to bring the attention back to the breath. As with most skills, the ability to do this gradually increases with practice.

Developing a generic skill of concentration in a meditation situation should generalize to a variety of situations in which concentration is an important component, particularly if the subjects/clients are encouraged to cultivate their concentration skills in these other situations. Anecdotal reports strongly support this, and many research studies suggest it is true (Murphy & Donovan, 1997). For example, meditation has been reported to improve concentration (Linden, 1973; Spanos et al., 1979) and to reduce insomnia (Schoicket et al., 1988). But what does not exist is a good body of controlled research showing the effects are specifically due to the cultivation of concentration, rather than to other meditation components, expectations, and so on.

When through concentration development a person reduces the agitation of the drunken monkey mind, the mind usually becomes more quiet and relaxed. Hence, in the world traditions, concentration meditations are often called tranquillity meditations. Instead of the mind being flooded with various perceptions, thoughts, and memories, there is a subjective sense of a decrease in mental contents and a decrease in their rate of movement through consciousness. This is accompanied by a sense of increased mental calmness and clarity. Since the mind and body are totally interconnected, relaxing the mind often relaxes the body; the reverse is also true. Biological relaxation is, by far, the most researched and best-documented meditation effect in the Western literature (Murphy & Donovan, 1997; Shapiro & Walsh, 1984; West, 1987), although, again, it has not yet been "proven" to be due to changes in a specific component, such as concentration. Some theorists have tended to reduce all of meditation to just another way to produce some generic relaxation response. But relaxation is just one possible effect of certain components of some types of meditation. Also, there are many more important effects of meditation than relaxation.

If meditation produces relaxation, then it can be used to reduce anxiety. And there is a substantial literature suggesting it is an effective treatment of anxiety for many people (Delmonte, 1985). The same would be expected for other undesirable emotional states such as anger. Also noted by Goleman (1971) and others, meditation often results in a natural counterconditioning with similarities to nonhierarchical desensitization. During meditation, affective material may enter consciousness. If the meditator remains relaxed, the affect may reduce by counterconditioning.

ATTENTION

Within NAMAP, concentration is a small part of the more general construct of attention, a major topic in learning and memory, sensation and perception, and therefore, cognitive science (Enns, 1990; Kinchla, 1992; LaBerge, 1990). Although some theorists define attention and concentration similarly, "attention" usually refers to a wider range of processes. In the dominant information processing theories, attention includes a set of processes for selecting information and allocating processing resources. Attention is involved in selecting, filtering, and funneling information. It is involved in deciding which processes and storages, of limited capacity, will be utilized in the processing of specific information. Thus, depending on one's theory or definition, attention may influence one or more (perhaps many) stages of the flow of information processing.

As delineated by Moray (1969), concentration is but one aspect of the varied functions of attention. The current attention literature terms that come closest to concentration are "focused attention," "controlled attention," "sustained attention," and "vigilance." However, these terms often refer more to the readiness and/or ability to detect the critical signal rather than the skill to maintain the desired focus of attention. Dember and Warm (1979, p. 148) define sustained attention as "the ability of observers to maintain their focus of attention and remain alert to stimuli over prolonged periods of time." They review a number of variables affecting sustained attention, including sensory modality of the signals, amplitude and duration of signals, signal-to-noise ratio and background event rate, temporal and/or spatial uncertainty of signal, and knowledge of results.

In the information processing literature, attention is often described as a prerequisite or opportunity for later conscious awareness. Sometimes attention is defined in terms of this awareness. But attention should not be confused with awareness, or concentration with mindfulness. Also, within the literature are many issues concerning unconscious processing and its possible influence on later conscious experience.

In Conjunctive Psychology, concentration is understood by integrating Western research on attention and Eastern research on cultivation of concentration. Western theories place concentration within other attentional factors and processes and thus help identify how these might interact with concentration. Western research identifies cues that attract attention or cause distraction. It suggests practical ways to structure the environment, the task, and the training to optimize attention and concentration. And it suggests the probable influence of a number of variables, such as context, arousal, and mental effort. Finally, a number of research procedures that have been used to study attention (e.g., dichotic listening, shadowing, Stroop effect) could be applied more specifically to concentration.

The major weakness in the Western literature is the inadequate understanding of the cultivation of concentration as a learned skill. Thus, practical interventions usually emphasize changing the environment or the task. Currently, the United States Navy is concerned about pilots' concentration. But all the research is devoted to changing the environment, such as aspects of the cockpit; no research investigates teaching pilots to have better concentration. A similar attitude is found in sports, where concentration is an important factor. In Western sports psychology, most research and theories about concentration are based on information-processing models; little research has been devoted to teaching athletes to have better concentration as a learned skill (Moran, 1996).

The major contribution of the Eastern psychologies is the recognition that one can develop concentration as a self-control skill. Thus, one can learn to maintain sustained attention despite distractions or associations. This mental skill has enormous therapeutic implications, and the Eastern literature provides a wealth of practical information on training concentration. The expression "behavior of the mind" helps remind us that concentration is a learned skill that everyone possesses in varying degrees in different situations.

ATTENTION DISORDERS

Probably the best-known attention disorder and currently the most widely studied childhood psychiatric disorder is what is currently called attention deficit hyperactivity disorder (ADHD). This traditionally involves hyperactivity, impulsiveness, and deficits in attention. Less well known is the related attention deficit disorder (ADD), which lacks the hyperactivity and impulsivity. Treatment of ADHD usually consists of some combination of drugs, behavior modification, and classroom management (Goldstein & Goldstein, 1990; Greenberg & Horn, 1991). Psychostimulant medication is used to help the child sustain attention, delay impulsive responses, control motor activity, and plan behavior. These drugs do not work in all cases or at all times with some cases, are not advisable with some children, and may produce side effects such as insomnia and decreased appetite. Behavior modification is used to deal with problematic behaviors and behavior deficits, in school and home, that result from the inattention and hyperactivity.

What is surprisingly missing in treatments of ADHD and ADD is systematic research on how such children and others can be taught self-control of their attention within the biological and social constraints. There are some games and treatment components to cultivate such concentration, but they are rare. Of the wide range of children diagnosed with ADHD, who could profit from learning concentration skills? And what is the best way to teach these children these skills?

"Self-focused attention" is a common problem across several clinical disorders (Ingram, 1990). It refers to an excessive amount of attention focused on the self, "an awareness of self-referent, internally generated information that stands in contrast to an awareness of externally generated information derived through sensory receptors" (Ingram, 1990, p. 156). Self-focused attention may be a cause or facilitator of a wide range of clinical problems. Again, the unanswered question is this: For which of these people would it be therapeutically useful to help them get control over the drunken monkey so that they can keep their minds from excessively running to contents that produce psychological problems? Self-focused attention would also be reduced by working with the other two behaviors of the mind discussed later: mindfulness and clinging.

There are many reports of anxious people having an "attentional bias," a tendency to attend disproportionately to cues related to potential threat and danger (Dalgleish & Watts, 1990). Perhaps anxiety causes this selective attention and/or the selective attention increases the anxiety. If anxiety is the cause of the attentional bias, then behavior modification to reduce the anxiety may reduce the bias (e.g., Lavy et al., 1993). If the attentional bias causes and/or increases the anxiety, then learning to control attention, as with concentration training, may be a way to reduce anxiety (e.g., Wells, 1990). A generic treatment program could contain both a concentration training component and an anxiety-reduction component, with the relative weights and sequencing of these components individualized.

Finally, consider the problem of unwanted thoughts, including some examples of "unintended thought" and "cognitive intrusions" such as obsessive thoughts, thoughts that disrupt or impair other behaviors (e.g., studying, listening), and thoughts that cause or accentuate anxiety, worry, anger, or pain. Such thoughts are very common in both clinical and nonclinical populations and people develop a variety of ways to try to deal with them, such as confronting them, suppressing them, or distracting themselves away from them (Freeston et al., 1991; Uleman & Bargh, 1989; Wegner & Pennebaker, 1993). However, most attempts to rid oneself of unwanted thoughts are not very effective. For example, thoughts that are temporarily suppressed often rebound back into consciousness (Rassin et al., 2000). And struggling with thoughts often empowers them and/or builds in additional associations. On the other hand, when people learn concentration as a cognitive self-control skill, they can easily stop most unwanted thoughts and/or stop the otherwise automatic chain of events that would flow from the thoughts (Murphy & Donovan, 1997). In some cases, stopping the thought is the best thing to do. In other cases, it is best to mindfully encounter the thoughts and keep the mind from running away.

Most people spend considerable time lost in thought and other contents of the mind. When various perceptions, memories, and thoughts arise, they are pulled into them and their reality is identified with them, particularly when the contents have great affect and/or personal significance. For example, Rachman (1997) suggests that what turns normal intrusive thoughts into obsessions is when the thoughts are misinterpreted as being personally significant, very important, revealing, threatening, or catastrophic. But with the development of concentration and mindfulness, a person gradually disidentifies with the contents of the mind and learns how to stand back and objectively observe the contents. This has two very strong implications for cognitive therapies. First, when a person is lost in the contents, it is much harder for her to objectively notice and observe the thoughts and beliefs that are important to the cognitive therapies. It is much easier to do from a more centered, quiet, disengaged position. Second, when someone is identified with contents of the mind, there is often resistance to change these contents. But when she observes the contents as just stuff of the mind and not who she is, there is usually less resistance to change the contents. For many people, it is often personally quite significant when they eventually disidentify with and disengage from the contents of their minds, even for a short period. From a psychoanalytic perspective, this objective distancing from contents of the mind might facilitate ego development (Boorstein, 1997).

There is considerable need and opportunity for research on when and how concentration learning might help some people with attention problems, such as those mentioned above. In addition, developing concentration helps people improve their overall enjoyment of living, such as learning how to leave the work at the office and how to stop and smell the roses.

BIOLOGY OF ATTENTION AND CONCENTRATION

To the extent that developing concentration quiets the mind and relaxes the mind and body, biological correlates would be what one would expect from relaxation (e.g., increased alpha and/or theta activity, lowered heart rate, reduced blood pressure, reduced muscle tension, and increased skin resistance). However, this is not a necessary result of concentration. It is possible to have a concentrated mind in nonrelaxed situations, such as sports.

For the broader topic of attention, there is a sizable literature of research and theories related to biological correlates and substrates of attention (Cohen, 1993; Parasuraman, 1998; van Zomeren & Brouwer, 1994). Cohen (1993) discusses a number of diseases that may impair sustained attention: multiple sclerosis, head trauma, Alzheimer's disease, Parkinson's disease, and brain neoplasms. Cohen points out that attention deficits are often core deficits in schizophrenia; and difficulty in concentration, often due to lack of "energy" or motivation, is a common symptom in affective disorders such as depression.

The term "attention" includes a wide variety of quite different yet overlapping processes. And each of these processes probably involves a number of different brain sites. Concentration probably involves the frontal cortex, parietal cortex, cingulate cortex, limbic system, and reticular formation, among other areas (Cohen, 1993).

MINDFULNESS

The second behavior of the mind is mindfulness, the active maximizing of the breadth and clarity of awareness. This definition of mindfulness is very similar to the way the term is used in Buddhism. But here the term is more intentional and behavioral, corresponding more to the cultivation of mindfulness in Buddhism.

When you become aware of a content of the mind, two things are arising simultaneously: the object of the awareness and the awareness itself. Because they arise at the same time, they are often confused and confounded. Thus, when NAMAP psychologists want to increase awareness, they usually do so by working with various potential objects of awareness. A great contribution of Buddhist psychology is the practical understanding that you can increase awareness directly, independent of the specific objects of awareness.

When you are consciously seeing, there is the visual object of perception and the awareness of the object. When you are consciously thinking, there are the thoughts and the awareness of the thoughts. The object of awareness (e.g., visual object, thought) is different from awareness itself. Thinking is not awareness! And we can work with this awareness directly, regardless of the specific objects of awareness. Mindfulness is the behavior of intentionally increasing the breadth and clarity of this awareness, the behavior of moving and sharpening focus within the field of consciousness. Sometimes mindfulness refers to maintaining ("maximizing") optimal breadth and clarity of awareness for that person at that time, rather than increasing breadth or clarity.

Breadth of awareness refers to the range of phenomena that do and could enter awareness. What is the person aware of? What is the person capable of being aware of? Increasing the breadth of awareness is a common goal of many disparate therapies. Psychoanalysis might attempt to bring into awareness repressed memories and perceptions. A primary goal of Gestalt therapy is to increase awareness of body, emotions, modes of thinking, how one treats oneself, and other behaviors. In behavior modification assessment and treatment, a client might learn how to be a better objective observer of his overt and covert behaviors. Clarity of awareness refers to the amount of distortion to the objects of awareness. When a perception or thought arises in someone's consciousness, how clearly does he perceive it instant by instant?

MINDFULNESS MEDITATION

Continuing the example of a meditator sitting quietly using the breath as the object of meditation: Whenever the mind leaves the breath, the meditator notes where it goes (mindfulness) and then gently and firmly brings the attention back to the breath (concentration). When the emphasis is on cultivating concentration, the person stresses developing one-pointedness on the breath. But there still should be a mindfulness component. However, when emphasis is on mindfulness, then the concentration component becomes secondary, sometimes minimal. For example, the meditator may simply let the mind go wherever it wants, but careful intention is given to noticing accurately whatever objects arise in consciousness. The essence of mindfulness training is simply noticing whatever arises in consciousness while minimizing the occurrence of and getting lost in related thoughts, reactions, and elaborations.

Many approaches exist for the cultivation of mindfulness during meditation, but the most comprehensive and developed is vipassana meditation from Theravada Buddhism (e.g., Goldstein, 1993; Goldstein & Kornfield, 1987; Hart, 1987; Mahasi Sayadaw, 1978, 1980). The vipassana literature includes many different sequences of instructions, all of which are intended to gradually increase the clarity and breadth of awareness, as one learns "to see" ("passana") "in a variety of ways" ("vi"). During sitting and walking meditation, the meditator learns to clearly perceive the flow of contents of the mind. Later the meditator gradually learns to perceive the behaviors of the mind and the dynamic processes one takes for one's "self." This leads to fundamental insights into the nature of one's reality and one's self. Hence, vipassana is often called insight meditation.

CULTIVATION OF MINDFULNESS

Although meditation is often a "simple" context within which to begin developing mindfulness, the important fact is that mindfulness can potentially be cultivated at any time in any situation! This point was strongly made by the Buddha in many ways. In a classic discourse (satipatthana), the Buddha suggested four "foundations" of mindfulness (Nyanaponika, 1962; Rahula, 1974; Silananda, 1990). These are four domains in which mindfulness can be cultivated: (1) body, including position, movement, breathing, biological cycles, and effects of stress and nutrition; (2) feelings, including pleasure, pain, and emotions; (3) mind, including the behaviors of the mind and defilements such as hatred and greed; and (4) mental factors, which refer to variables and characteristics of the mind specifically related to the development of psychospiritual freedom or enlightenment. There is, of course, overlap among these categories and other ways to categorize domains of mindfulness.

Traditionally, the most common forms for cultivating mindfulness are sitting and walking meditations, but these forms are best for only some people. Now, a wider range of forms and practices is being developed (Hanh, 1975; Tart, 1990) as well as specific mindfulness questionnaires (DeMaria & Mikulas, 1991; Mikulas, 1990). In therapy situations, what is critical is being able to develop individualized forms geared toward the interests and needs of specific clients. For example, for a person with eating problems we would develop mindfulness exercises related to the act of eating and corresponding cravings and emotions. For a person with a lot of anxiety, we would develop specific mindfulness exercises related to relevant feelings and thoughts.

After an appropriate form for mindfulness training has been established, it is necessary to reinforce the behavior itself. Many people enjoy cultivating mindfulness with personalized exercises (as opposed to the unpleasant struggle many have in trying to cultivate concentration). Shaping is, of course, critical, as can be seen in the vipassana programs. Ideally, the client recognizes and accepts where he is and then gradually and systematically increases breadth and clarity of awareness. Some of the new areas that awareness moves into may be psychologically troubling. Gradually moving into these areas while remaining calm and centered will reduce the negative affect. In some cases, the client needs the support and guidance of the therapist for moving into problem areas.

Establishing discriminative stimuli for the behavior of mindfulness can be helpful. These are stimuli that cue the person to be mindful. It might be a sign on the refrigerator or mirror, a ring or bracelet, or a particular type of feeling or thought. The possibilities are endless and become more and more subtle.

Another important variable, often given inadequate attention, is a person's "attitude" toward mindfulness, the mental set in which he approaches developing mindfulness. Mentioned above in terms of meditation attitude, this includes a welcoming openness to experience, choiceless awareness, a contentment to be in the here and now, a persistence to perceive clearly, and a gradually developing sense of equanimity in which the person is equally happy with and interested in whatever arises in his consciousness.

The three behaviors of the mind (concentration, mindfulness, clinging) are all totally interrelated and often confused with each other. A change in one behavior will generally produce a change in the others. Hence, in practical situations, it is often most effective to work with more than one behavior at a time. For example, improving concentration will generally facilitate mindfulness. If the drunken monkey is running wildly about, it is difficult to clearly perceive everywhere it goes. As the mind is calmed and one-pointedness increased, one can more clearly perceive what arises in consciousness. Conversely, increasing mindfulness helps in cultivating concentration, for one of the things the person becomes mindful of is how concentrated his mind is.

SELF-CONTROL

The act of self-control involves awareness that something must be done, plus what you do. First you are aware of the presence of a less preferred behavior and/or a sequence of events leading to a less preferred behavior. Then you utilize some intervention strategy to reduce the less preferred behavior and/or to increase a desired alternative.

Beth Hardcastle developed a questionnaire for impulsive middle school children. The questionnaire assessed awareness of cues and knowledge of strategies relative to self-control of impulsive behavior. One finding of importance was that some children had the necessary self-control intervention skills but were not aware of becoming impulsive until it was too late. Other children were aware of being in a situation where undesired impulsive behaviors were likely, but they did not have the intervention skills to avoid the behaviors. Traditionally, these two groups of children would be treated similarly. But when looked at more closely, it is clear that for one group, emphasizing mindfulness training is desirable, and for the other, learning intervention skills is best.

Behavior modification has a rich literature of powerful techniques to contribute to the intervention component of self-control, but is quite weak in terms of the awareness component (Ladouceur & Mercier, 1984). Adding mindfulness training is often the most direct and effective way to increase the awareness component. Sometimes this may be a sufficient treatment in itself. If the person has the necessary intervention skill and is motivated to utilize it, then simply increasing awareness of when to do it may be sufficient. In most cases, however, we would also want to help the person acquire or develop the intervention strategy.

Very important and largely unrecognized is the fact that with mindfulness training we can move the awareness earlier and earlier in the chain of events, making self-control easier and giving the person more freedom and choice. Consider a person who has trouble controlling anger (or anxiety, or . . .). He finds himself caught up in angry thoughts and feelings before he sees them coming on. At this point it may be difficult to get out of the anger, and his mind may be justifying why it is appropriate to be angry in this situation. Later, with mindfulness training he learns to be aware when he starts to feel angry and when angry thoughts start to occur. At this point it is much easier for him to apply a self-control intervention and stop the anger from developing. With more mindfulness training he learns to be aware of when he is predisposed toward anger, and here it is quite easy to prevent the anger.

Psychoanalysis

There are many similarities between psychoanalysis and mindfulness meditation, and thus many ways they might be combined (e.g., Boorstein, 1997). Both mindfulness and psychodynamic inquiry, such as free association, encourage clients to open their conscious minds to new or repressed material and to actively notice what arises. In some cases, clients are encouraged to immerse themselves in particular contents of the mind, such as a memory, for therapeutic reasons (e.g., extinction of emotional affect). Here a form of contemplative meditation might be helpful. In other cases, clients are encouraged to mindfully witness the content (e.g., memory) from a here-and-now stance. Thus, instead of being immersed and lost in the memory, the client objectively observes the memory as mental activity occurring in the present. This gives her some distance from the memory, reduces its affect, and facilitates cognitive change. When clients should immerse in the contents and when they should mindfully disengage is an important clinical issue (Cortright, 1997). Both mindfulness and psychoanalysis lead to clients' insights, which may create opportunities for additional therapeutic work.

A major difference between traditional mindfulness training and psychoanalysis is that in psychoanalysis the therapist is more involved with the client during consciousness expansion: interacting with the client, encouraging and guiding the client, and providing maps of the territory. Also, in psychoanalysis, the client is usually encouraged to engage and work through the content that arises, rather than just notice it as in most mindfulness training. And in psychoanalysis, it is usually assumed that the relationship between therapist and client is a potentially rich source of material to be mindful of and work with.

Clinging

A third behavior of the mind is clinging, the tendency of the mind to grasp for and cling to certain contents of the mind, assumptions about self and reality, and personal frames of references. Of all the different potential contents of the mind and ways of constructing one's personal reality, the mind will cling to some at the expense of others. This includes certain perceptions, rituals, expectancies, opinions, images of the self, and models of reality. Following Indian yogic psychology, the result of this clinging will be called an attachment. The term "addiction" could be used instead of "attachment," but "attachment" is cleaner. Note this is different from the psychodynamic use of the term "attachment," which refers to interpersonal bonding, usually early in life, such as between an infant and the mother (Bowlby, 1984). This psychodynamic attachment may be a special case of the more general type of attachment discussed here.

Attachments result in psychological inertia, a resistance to change, even when the change would make the person's life more effective and happier. A person may become very attached to a behavior because it has become part of his routine and/or the way he defines himself. Then he might resist changing this ritual behavior. Similarly, it is common for a person to continually do something that is wrong, stupid, or self-defeating in order to justify having been doing it for so long and/or as part of not seeing it as it really is. Thus attachments are barriers to personal and transpersonal growth and tend to keep people stuck in past behavior patterns and perceptions of self and reality (Keyes, 1975; Maul & Maul, 1983).

A very broad and central construct in Buddhist psychology is "dukkha" (Claxton, 1992; Rahula, 1974), which is usually translated as "suffering," but actually means something closer to "unsatisfactoriness." Dukkha includes most of what would be called "anxiety" in Western psychology, including behavioral, personal, and existential forms of anxiety. But dukkha includes much more and hence is an important construct when integrating Eastern and Western psychologies.

A common form of dukkha is a sense of personal and/or spiritual unsatisfactoriness, possibly including the feeling that things are not quite right, the sense that real happiness is continually out of reach, and/or the conviction that one can't get free. Dukkha is apparent when people collect stuff (e.g., possessions, money, power, fame) in a generally futile quest for happiness or peace of mind. Dukkha is often part of the motivation that drives people to religion, spirituality, science, psychology, and other possible cures.

A very profound basis of Buddhist psychology is the Four Noble Truths (Mikulas, 1978b; Rahula, 1974). The first noble truth asserts the widespread prevalence of dukkha. The second noble truth asserts that the cause of dukkha is the craving and clinging of the mind. One common reason that clinging causes dukkha is that everything changes. If an individual is attached to her youth, the specifics of a relationship, or a particular self-image, she will probably suffer when these change. There is less dukkha if one accepts and enjoys different ages, lets relationships evolve, and has a less rigid sense of "self." The third noble truth asserts that one can reduce dukkha by reducing the craving that leads to clinging. And the fourth noble truth outlines the Buddhist way for reducing craving, the Eightfold Path (Das, 1997, Rahula, 1974).

The grasping and clinging of the second Noble Truth is elaborated on in the law of dependent origination discussed earlier (Buddhadasa, 1992; Nyanatiloka, 1971). First comes "contact," awareness of a sensation. This leads to "feeling," discerning whether the sensation is positive, negative, or neutral. Then comes "craving," possible motivation to consume or escape. Next is "grasping," clinging and attachments to some objects and avoidance of others. And this leads to "becoming," the results of clinging and attachments, discussed below. Vipassana therapy involves cultivating mindfulness backward through the chain to craving, perhaps to feeling. Then a self-control skill is used to break the sequence.

As discussed earlier, there is considerable confusion between behaviors of the mind and contents of the mind. Relative to clinging, an important point is that clinging is always problematical, even though what one clings to may or may not be problematical. Clinging always produces undesirable results, such as the psychological effects discussed below, dukkha, and resistance to personal and transpersonal growth. On the other hand, what a person is attached to may be judged desirable or not, according to many other criteria, including practical, psychological, ethical, and legal considerations. For example, money in itself is not "good" or "bad," but being attached to money, so that it impairs relationships with other people and causes excessive anxiety, is problematical. There is a common expression, "Money is the root of all evil." But the biblical quotation from which this probably came is "The love of money is the root of all evil" (I Timothy 6:10).

RESULTS OF CLINGING

Clinging and attachments are most easily recognized and researched in terms of their effects. Three of the most common psychological effects are distortion of perception, impairment in thinking, and undesired emotions. Our attachments influence what we attend to, what gets into consciousness, and the specifics of the perception. Our thinking is limited and impaired by clinging to assumptions, following the same paths of reasoning, and fearing that we will be "wrong." And when our craving is not fulfilled in the way our attachments demand, we may get anxious, angry, or jealous.

These types of effects, and proposed related processes, are described in many NAMAP psychological theories, including psychodynamic defense mechanisms, cognitive dissonance theory, the "new look" in perception, and schemas in cognitive psychology. In all these, we see how processes similar to clinging distort perception, impair thinking, and elicit undesired emotions. The Western psychological literature, including clinical psychology, social psychology, perception, and cognition, are filled with research and theories related to clinging. Samples are given next.

A very common result of clinging and attachments is the elicitation of undesired emotions such as anxiety, fear, worry, sadness, jealousy, frustration, disappointment, anger, irritation, or resentment, to name just a few. "Undesired" here means unpleasant, unwanted, destructive, impairing thinking and perception, creating barriers, closing the heart, and limiting personal/transpersonal growth. Observing, and perhaps measuring, undesired emotions is one of the easiest ways to detect attachments for research, therapy, and personal/transpersonal work. An attachment is often an emotion-backed demand, expectation, or model that elicits an undesired emotion if not satisfied (Keyes, 1975). If Cindy demands that her child act in a specific way and he doesn't, Cindy may get mad. If Michelle expects a social evening to progress in a certain way and it doesn't, Michelle may get irritated or disappointed. If Jeff has a model of what the ideal boss should be like and she isn't like that, then Jeff may feel frustration and resentment.

People compare their perception of reality (world, other people, self, etc.) with their models and expectations of how they think reality should be and/or how they wish it to be. If the discrepancy is great enough, the people will get upset. Note that using the discrepancy to influence and guide future behavior is a natural and appropriate feedback mechanism, but the undesired emotion that results from such a discrepancy is unnecessary and unwanted for optimal living and is usually a sign of an attachment. In addition, the undesired emotion and correlated impaired thinking and perceiving all may hamper effective behavior for reducing the discrepancy. Jim's daughter is not living the way Jim thinks she should, which upsets Jim and impairs his thinking, which then makes him less effective at influencing her toward what Jim thinks is right, which then upsets Jim, and the circle continues.

This type of emotional response to discrepancies between perceived reality and attached models and expectations is very common; many people can quickly learn to see many examples each day. It also underlies many issues that helpers will often encounter. Because the models and expectations frequently include images and concepts of the "self," a domain of many attachments, the discrepancies are often particularly personal and threatening.

One way of reducing this type of anxiety is through self-deception, the act of lying to yourself and/or denying yourself certain information (Lockard & Paulhus, 1988). In some cases, this self-deception may have psychological benefits, affecting self-esteem, motivation, and social relations (cf. Taylor, 1989). Goleman (1985) suggests that the mind protects itself against anxiety by diminishing awareness, creating a zone of blocked attention and self-deception. He postulates that endorphins may be the agents that numb sensations of pain and dim attention.

Similar are the excuses and attributions that people devise. People will delude themselves about causes of events and behaviors in order to reduce or avoid perceived discrepancies related to attached views of self and control (Snyder & Higgins, 1988). This is similar to some examples of "hindsight" where people use current knowledge to alter memories or past beliefs about the outcome of some event (Hawkins & Hastie, 1990). Knowing the outcome of an event, a person now believes I "knew all along" it would turn out this way. Attachments might be related to someone's image of herself as a knower of such events and/or to the personal investment she has in particular outcomes.

Kenny and DePaulo (1993) suggest that the way people determine how others view them is based more on their own self-perceptions than on feedback they receive from others. In addition, people often overestimate the amount of consistency in others' views of them. These inaccurate perceptions can impair developing interpersonal relationships. Social perceptions and beliefs may be strengthened through dynamics such as self-fulfilling prophecies, where one person's expectancies about a second person lead the second person to act in ways that confirm these expectancies (Jones, 1986; Jussim, 1986).

Clinging "simplifies" the world and thus results in less need for thinking and decision making. Clinging to assumptions often impairs thinking when the assumption is inaccurate or limited. Clinically, clinging to assumptions often produces a variety of personal and interpersonal problems. Common examples include clinging to assumptions about oneself (e.g., self-concept), other people (e.g., opposite gender), "necessary" aspects of social relationships (e.g., marriage, boss, and subordinate), what is appropriately assertive (as opposed to nonassertive or aggressive), "optimal" sexual intercourse (e.g., male as initiator, simultaneous orgasm), and the potential and desirability for change in oneself and others. Therapy often consists of identifying such assumptions and perhaps challenging and/or changing them.

Questioning assumptions has led to many small and great intellectual discoveries. Considering alternatives to the parallel postulate led to non-Euclidean geometries. One of these geometries plus questioning the assumptions about the relative/absolute speed of light set the stage for Einstein's theory of relativity. Thus, most programs designed to increase creativity and improve thinking generally encourage challenging assumptions and thinking in new ways (e.g., Adams, 1986; de Bono 1970, 1982). Currently, the research on the effectiveness of such approaches has generated mixed results (Weisberg, 1993), but the potential implications for therapy and education are very great. Similarly, attachments about the outcome of thinking may impair the thinking. For example, when reasoning, people are more likely to arrive at conclusions they want to arrive at, particularly if they can construct reasonable justifications for the conclusions (Kunda, 1990).

Finally, emotions caused by attachments often impair thinking. A student with test anxiety misses things on a test that he knew before and after the test. A person who is angry because of an interpersonal conflict may not think as clearly as usual about the best way to resolve the conflict.

REDUCING ATTACHMENTS

When reducing attachments, three common important components are attitude, awareness, and action. Attitude is the mental set in which an individual approaches attachments and includes the components of meditation attitude. In addition, it includes a person's attitude toward discovering attachments. If it is disturbing or unpleasant to become aware of an attachment, then he will tend not to become aware of them. On the other hand, if he takes delight in discovering attachments, appreciating the opportunity to identify and perhaps overcome a personal barrier, then he will gradually notice more and more attachments. Through a change in values, there is a switch from a punishment contingency to a reinforcement contingency.

The second component in attachment work is awareness, mindfulness of the effects, dynamics, and eliciting stimuli of attachments. Usually, at first the effects are easier to notice and they become discriminative stimuli for cultivating mindfulness of other aspects of attachments, clinging, and craving. The third component of attachment work is action, what a person does when an attachment is observed. This could be one of a very diverse set of possible actions, including behavior modification self-control skills, meditation-based skills, and psychospiritual practices.

A conceptual scheme for categorizing attachments can sometimes help in identifying and thinking about attachments. For example, in yogic psychology it is suggested that most attachments are related to security, sensation, and/or power, corresponding to the first three chakras, discussed later (Rama et al., 1976). Thus, when you are upset, you notice and reflect on what attachments are at work and how they relate to security, sensation, and/or power (cf. Keyes, 1975; Mikulas, 1987). An attachment log is often helpful.

Security attachments, generating fear, worry, or paranoia, might center on such things as possessions, home, relationships, social roles, self-concept, other's opinions of us, and being wrong. Sensation attachments relate to craving for sensory pleasure and greater complexity, fleeing from boredom and sameness, and sex in the broadest sense. Power attachments may be related to issues of will, domination and submission, social-political influence, prestige, pride, and energy.

The three behaviors of the mind are all intertwined; changes in one result in or facilitate changes in the others. For example, quieting the mind and increasing mindfulness make it easier to notice attachments and craving, to notice them earlier and earlier, and to let go of them. Reducing attachments removes obstacles to mindfulness and reduces upsetting mental factors that impair the mind's tranquillity.

INTEGRATIVE HELPERS

It is very important that, over many years, integrative helpers spend considerable time and attention to working with themselves, with the above three behaviors of the mind! This point cannot be overemphasized. An integrative helper must eventually have many stories of personal adventures with the drunken monkey. The contents of the mind, such as what one is mindful of or attached to, will naturally vary among people; but the behaviors of the mind are universal. Potentially, in any situation, one can be mindful of and working with one or more of the behaviors. Integrative helpers structure their time and activities for such work, in forms that are personally useful and/or fun.

A sufficient reason for helpers to work with their own behaviors of the mind is that it will improve their lives. This, in turn, will make them better helpers. As the helpers' perceptions clear, minds quiet, and attachments reduce, they can be better models and friends to their clients.

A second reason for helpers to work with their behaviors is that it will improve the interpersonal helping skills advocated by various theorists, including those who favor the humanistic approaches. Quieting the mind and increasing mindfulness make the helper a better and more objective observer of client and self. This is related to the general issue of training of observational skills, an important but neglected topic in NAMAP (cf. Boice, 1983). For many helpers, during initial sessions with the clients the drunken monkeys are running about. Rather than optimally hearing the client, the helper's mind is filled with reactions, associations, labeling and categorizing, and premature treatment planning. This monkey business distorts her perception and impairs her thinking about the client. By quieting the mind, the helper listens better and is more empathic. Empathy is further increased when the helper becomes more mindful of the client and herself and becomes aware of the effects of her own attachments. She learns how to disengage from her own personal melodrama and to see, feel, and think as much as possible from the client's perspective. There is some research evidence that meditation can increase empathy (e.g., Lesh, 1970; Schuster, 1979).

The third reason for helpers to work with their own behaviors of the mind is that this is usually the best way to learn about these behaviors. It makes the helpers more effective at helping clients with their mind behaviors. Very important, as helpers become more and more knowledgeable about behaviors of the mind, they can better develop individualized forms for clients' mental training and interface this training with other parts of the treatment program.

SUMMARY

Behaviors of the mind are the processes that select and construct the contents of the mind and that provide awareness of these contents. Three such behaviors are concentration, mindfulness, and clinging.

Concentration is the learned control of focusing one's attention. Cultivating concentration can enhance a person's ability to study, listen, enjoy sensory experiences, and control the contents of the mind. Developing concentration also quiets and relaxes the mind, which then relaxes the body.

Mindfulness is the active maximizing of the breadth and clarity of awareness. One learns to become aware of more things and perceive them more clearly. Cultivating mindfulness can potentially improve anything that a person does, and is particularly important for optimal self-control.

Clinging refers to the tendency of the mind to grasp for and cling to certain contents of consciousness and/or personal frames of reference. Clinging may result in resistance to change, distortion of perception, impaired thinking, and/or negative emotions.

Behaviors of the mind can be altered with behavior modification, and can be studied behaviorally and neurophysiologically. The construct of behaviors of the mind is unique to Conjunctive Psychology, a complementary alternative to information processing models, a next logical step for cognitive behavior therapists, and heuristic in interfacing Eastern and Western psychologies. For example, all the world's major forms of meditation involve cultivating concentration and/or mindfulness.

Because the behaviors of the mind are always present, they can potentially be cultivated in any situation and have important applications for all settings. Thus, working with these behaviors can be an important part of programs in psychology, health, education, sports, arts, and personal/spiritual growth.

It is critical for integrative helpers to work with their own behaviors of the mind. This will significantly improve their lives, make them more effective helpers, and enhance their ability to help others work with behaviors of the mind.

AUTHOR'S REFLECTIONS

I have been heavily involved in meditation for several decades, as a student, practitioner, teacher, and researcher. I have been fortunate to have had many good teachers, including my students. In my occasional role as a teacher, I have worked with individuals, college classes, professional workshops, and free community classes with hundreds of people. On an international level, I have been involved with individuals and groups concerned with exploring how meditation can be used to enhance heath and psychological well-being (e.g., Kaku, 2000). From this, I have come to realize and appreciate why, around the world and across the centuries, meditation has been the most recommended practice for improving body, mind, and spirit.

Although meditation can be learned from books (Bodian, 1999; LeShan, 1974), it is usually best to learn it from a teacher. One reason is that meditation, like most powerful practices, is not right for everyone, and can hurt some people.

Fifty years ago, there was little traditional meditation in the United States. Now it is very common, and there are good teachers and centers representing all the major traditions. However, in addition, much of what is called "meditation," I would classify otherwise, such as guided imagery.

Despite the power and popularity of meditation, it is slow coming into NAMAP. For example, every year I am sent at least a dozen introductory psychology texts, almost all of which contain the same basic NAMAP overview. Most of them will have just a couple of paragraphs on meditation, and almost all describe it as a form of relaxation, often in the context of stress reduction. But meditation is much more than that!

One problem with meditation, for practitioners and for NAMAP understanding, is confusing the different components of meditation (form, object, attitude, behavior of mind). Practitioners can get caught up in the form or object and lose sight of the real purpose of meditation. Or, people who wish to learn what meditation is may have trouble seeing past the many forms and objects to the essence of the practice.

My solution to this is to clearly specify and differentiate the four components, one of which is the behaviors of the mind being cultivated: concentration and/or mindfulness. Concentration and mindfulness can then be researched without the usual confounding with form and object. More important is the realization that concentration and mindfulness can be cultivated during any activity, not just meditation. This has significant implications for the integrative helper, as discussed in the chapter.

The concept of attachments, that result from the clinging behavior of the mind, is a very heuristic conceptualization. It is easy to understand, which makes it effective in many applied situations, including therapy, personal growth, and spiritual practice. It is a concept that incorporates a wide range of psychological processes and issues, which gives it frequent applicability and makes it a useful construct for integrating psychologies. And there is a general practical strategy for dealing with most attachments, although the particulars of the strategy will vary tremendously.

A beauty of attachments is that everyone has many opportunities every day to observe and work with them. A very common example is for someone to become upset when reality does not match a model or expectation of how reality should be. Learning how to deal with simple attachments prepares the person for working with the more difficult ones.

If you seriously want to improve your life significantly, then quiet your mind, increase mindfulness, and reduce attachments. I will later add opening the heart to this list.

THOUGHT QUESTIONS

1. For a hypothetical case, describe how you assessed the person's thoughts and how these thoughts related to other behaviors.
(2.) How does the object of awareness differ from awareness itself?
3. How does concentration differ from mindfulness? Why are they often confused?
4. Sit quietly for five minutes, with eyes closed and your attention on your breath going in and out of your nose (or mouth, if necessary). Try to keep your attention on your breath. What did you learn?
5. Imagine, in detail, a big lion. Now, for five minutes try not to think of a lion. What did you learn?
6. What motivates the drunken monkey?
7. What does it mean in Buddhist psychology to say almost everyone has ADHD?
8. For a hypothetical case of a child classified as ADHD, describe how developing concentration could be part of the treatment program. Be specific.
9. When developing a questionnaire to assess overall concentration and mindfulness, give three sample questions for each.
(10.) How can fading and shaping be applied to developing concentration and mindfulness?
(11.) Describe a hypothetical case in which developing mindfulness is sufficient therapy.
(12.) Before reading this chapter, what notions did you have about meditation? What did this word mean to you? How have your views changed?
13. Give three personal examples showing that clinging produces dukkha.
14. Give three examples in which the object of clinging is desirable, but the clinging is causing problems.
(15.) Give a clinical example of attachments and what the therapist might do to bring about change.
16. For at least a week, keep an attachment log. Each day, write down at least two examples of attachments that caused distorted perception, impaired thinking, and/or undesired emotions. How did you notice the attachment? What did you do about it? Classify the attachments according to the first three chakras. What are you learning about your personal attachments?
17. How do the three behaviors of the mind relate to sports and art?
18. Give concrete examples for how the three behaviors of the mind influence each other.
19. In Buddhist psychology, the seven factors of the enlightened mind are concentration, mindfulness, investigation, effort, interest, calm, and equanimity. Describe how cultivating the last five helps the first two.

four

PERSONAL LEVEL

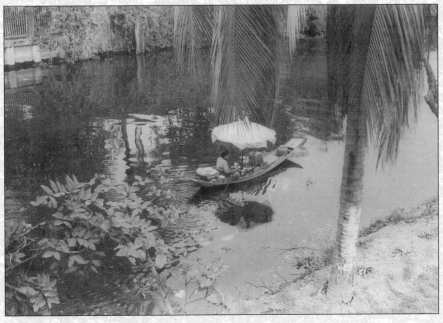

Photo by Benita Mikulas

Conscious Personal Reality

Although all levels of being are totally intertwined, it is heuristic to make distinctions among levels. Consciousness is an important distinguishing feature. One does not need the construct of consciousness to adequately explain the inner dynamics of the biological level or the behavioral level. Many behaviorists actively avoid any reference to consciousness. But consciousness is a defining feature of the personal level and the transpersonal level. The personal level is concerned with individual consciousness; the transpersonal level is concerned with consciousness as a field and a property of the fundamental ground.

A second distinguishing feature of the personal level is the sense of self and the interrelated sense of will. One is conscious of a sense of self that seems to be the observer in the conscious reality. And this self periodically, through an act of will, seems to be the agent of some behaviors. The conscious reality the self lives in is unique to the individual and influenced by many variables, such as culture. Hence, the personal level is defined as the domain of the conscious, self-centered, personal reality.

Consciousness

The "mind-body problem" is a persistent issue in Western philosophy and is probably unresolvable by current philosophical methods. The "body" is the unthinking, observable substance that constitutes the form of a person. The "mind," on the other hand, has no substance or form and is conscious and thinks. The mind-body problem is the question of how two entities as different as mind and body can influence each other (Globus et al., 1976). Various "solutions" include reducing one to the other, suggesting they run in parallel and don't interact, and describing how one might influence the other. For example, Descartes advocated a dualism in which mind and body are direct and complete opposites but interact through the pineal gland. Skinner and most cognitive scientists advocate a form of monism in which mind and body are simply two aspects of the same thing. Currently, the major Western version of the mind-body problem is how consciousness relates to the brain (Burns, 1990). Within NAMAP, consciousness is generally seen as a product or emergent property of the brain; consciousness comes from the brain. Interestingly, the exact opposite position is suggested in Vedanta (the major philosophy of Hinduism) and in the descriptions of mystics of all traditions. Here it is proposed that consciousness, as an aspect of the fundamental ground, comes first; and all objects, including the brain, arise out of consciousness.

In the mindfulness meditation practices of vipassana, one observes for oneself the interaction between mind (nama) and body (rupa). The Insight Meditation Society defines vipassana/insight meditation as "the moment-to-moment investigation of the mind/body process through calm and focused awareness." When one intends to move or thinks about moving, how does one's body respond and prepare? When one has an emotional perception or memory, what specifically does the body do? When one has a psychological or spiritual insight, how does that manifest in the body? What exactly are the effects of quieting the mind on the body? Conversely, how does body movement influence the contents and mood of the mind? How does breathing affect the nature and state of consciousness? How do body sensations, such as pain, influence the state and contents of the mind?

Within NAMAP, consciousness as an explanatory variable and topic of research fell into disrepute during the first half of the 20th century, then reemerged as a popular topic in the second half (Farthing, 1992; Hunt, 1995; Ornstein 1986; Pelletier, 1978; Wallace & Fisher, 1999). Relatedly, interest in the philosophy of consciousness also recently mushroomed in popularity (Block et al., 1997). Common topics in the Western psychology of consciousness include consciousness and the brain, conscious versus unconscious processing, possible relationships to quantum physics and chaos theory, parapsychology, evolution of consciousness, and different states and levels of consciousness.

PERSONAL REALITY

Study of consciousness at the personal level focuses on the individual's conscious experiences, the personal reality. The critical point is that this is a learned reality, unique to the individual, and affected by motivation (Strauch, 1989). How learning and motivation affect one's perceived reality is a very complex topic that draws from many areas of psychology, including perception (Gregory, 1966), social psychology (O'Brien & Kollock, 1997), constructivism (Neimeyer, 1993; Rosen & Kuehlwein, 1996; Winter, 1992), clinical psychology, and attachment research. Here are a few pieces of this vast area.

For discussion sake, assume the philosophical position of "realism," that there is an external world that exists independent of our minds. One's experience of this world is through the senses at the biological level, sometimes aided by technology (e.g., glasses, telescope). But there are extraordinary differences between sensation at the biological level and conscious perception at the personal level. Hearing at the biological level involves sound waves moving the eardrum and motion of fluid in the inner ear. But this is not what is perceived at the personal level. Instead, there are voices and music seeming to come from specific sources.

Consider visual depth perception. At the biological level, there are photons/light waves striking the retina, basically a two-dimensional surface. This results in neural activity influenced by the behaviors of perception at the behavioral level. Then, for most people, there arises in consciousness a colored three-dimensional world. How did two dimensional input of light (electromagnetic radiation) from objects that are primarily empty space result in consciousness of a three-dimensional world of solid objects? Research in perception has identified the cues that are used in constructing a sense of depth (Dember & Warm, 1979). But it is the learning that is important here. For example, if the image of a dog grows in size on your retina, you don't see a dog getting bigger; you see the dog moving closer. You have learned that dogs do not rapidly change in size, and your perception is guided by this learning. If the image on your retina is of one person's head on top of another, you don't see a two-headed person. You see one person behind another. Although utilization of depth cues at the behavioral level is usually associated with, and confounded with, a conscious perception of three dimensions, this is not always so. Bob was an example (Mikulas, 1996a). As a child, he realized he had no depth perception but saw the world as two-dimensional. He was impaired in throwing and catching. He would not jump down from something because he could not tell how far it was to the ground. As a young professional, he could not join his friends in learning to fly because he could not judge visually whether he was 10 or 100 feet off the ground. All this time, his brain used dimensional cues for practical activity, but the lack of subjective dimensionality created impairments. At the age of 45, Bob was sitting in the mountains of North Carolina smoking marijuana when suddenly he became aware of seeing three-dimensionally. He was in a place of spectacular views, beautiful hills of varying sizes in sequence extending over considerable distance. People with normal vision in such a place are often impressed by a sense of greater dimensionality. In addition, a common result of using marijuana is an increased sense of dimensionality. For awhile, the experience of dimensionality came and went. When it was not there, Bob could usually call it up by trying to see depth. Gradually, dimensionality became usual, but he could still choose to see things in two dimensions. However, after one year, Bob perceived only three-dimensionally and could no longer see otherwise.

Our culture influences our visual perception (Deregowski, 1980; Segall et al., 1966). The culture provides things to perceive and reinforces different types of discrimination among the objects. Eskimos learn to perceive different types of snow, some Filipinos learn to perceive different varieties of rice, and American teenage boys often are able to make fine distinctions among cars. The culture also provides the language that influences some combination of perception, memory, and thinking, in ways that are difficult to separate (Hardin & Banaji, 1993; Hunt & Agnoli, 1991).

For example, in English the world is divided into objects (nouns), actions and processes (verbs), and qualifiers (adjectives and adverbs). Thus, an English-speaking person's worldview has object-action duality. When we see apples on a tree, we perceive/think in terms of a tree producing apples, as opposed, for example, to a tree "appling." When we see a tree swaying about, we perceive/think in terms of a wind blowing the tree. If there is no obvious subject, we insert "it," as in "it" is raining. We make objects out of events, such as day, summer, and thunder. In addition to grammatical effects, there are the many effects of vocabulary. Among the languages of the Native Americans there is no word for "art"; for everything is art and therefore needs no special term. How does our conceptualizing art into something special create an experiential division between art and commonplace experiences?

As a result of language learning and discrimination learning, we develop categories or schemas for information processing. This is necessary for practical and efficient interacting with the world. We respond to objects based on how they are categorized, rather than dealing with them as unique objects. Unfortunately, this can result in perceptual distortion when disparate sensations are forced into the same category. Consider a person who has considerable experience with American playing cards, with red hearts and black spades. If this person is quickly shown a red queen of spades, he will probably perceive it as a black queen of spades or red queen of hearts, corresponding to his card categories. In some cases, there will be a compromise reaction and he might perceive a purple queen of spades (Bruner & Postman, 1949). Social psychology is filled with examples of peoples' misperceptions based on categories (e.g., Cohen, 1981). This includes misperceptions based on race, gender, nationality, and religion.

Attachments, discussed in the last chapter, often influence or distort perception. One person with security attachments perceives threats that are not there. Another person with sensation attachments sees many people in terms of potential sexual partners, thus overlooking more important characteristics in these and other people. Two people with opposite political attachments may have very different and contradictory perceptions of the same political talk.

Motivation affects perception in many ways. Of all the things we can attend to, we focus on those that are most important in some way (selective attention). Some of these important things may be easier to perceive because they are important (perceptual vigilance). On the other hand, if perceiving something will cause us anxiety, then the perception may be distorted or kept out of consciousness (perceptual defense, avoidance conditioning).

So far the discussion has focused on perception, but all the major points also apply to memory (cf. Neath, 1998; Schacter, 1996). Calling up a memory is rarely the simple playback of a recorded experience. Rather, often a memory is constructed from pieces of information, filling in gaps based on past learning, and altering parts based on motivation and beliefs. Between the neurophysiological correlates of memory at the biological level and the constructed conscious memory at the personal level, the construction process is heavily influenced by the same factors that influence perception, including language, categories/schemas, attachments, and motivation.

Memories can be altered and false memories implanted through standard persuasion techniques, such as suggestion and guided probing (Neath, 1998; Schacter et al., 1995). This might be done, intentionally or not, by a therapist, hypnotist, magician, attorney, political propagandist, or cult leader. For example, consider an eyewitness of a traffic accident who is asked "Was the car stopped at the stop sign?" Although it was actually a yield sign, as a result of the question, the witness may later remember a stop sign (Loftus et al., 1978). During the 1980s in the United States, there was a rash of cases in which therapists and ministers implanted false memories in people, memories related to being abused as children. Child psychologist Piaget once told of his earliest memory, almost being abducted from his baby carriage when he was two years old. Piaget could remember many details of the event: the intervention by his nurse, resulting scratches on the nurse's face, and a policeman chasing the villain. Years later, the nurse admitted having made up the whole story.

Imagine guards who work at the gates of Personal Reality. Their main job is to stop potential intruders (perceptions, memories, thoughts) that might cause trouble if let in. The two main, often related, sources of trouble are too much affect (such as anxiety, anger, or sorrow) and too much of a challenge to the person's belief about reality and self. Some would-be intruders are simply stopped; others are allowed in after they are changed into more acceptable members of the realm. Sometimes the guards are simply overwhelmed by an intruder, who rushes in. Sometimes the guards fall asleep or are drugged. And sometimes the guards are attacked from within the realm with demands to open the gates more. The behavior of the guards can be described in terms of psychodynamic defense mechanisms, cognitive balance theories such as cognitive dissonance theory, behavioral escape and avoidance learning, schemas, and attachments. There are, of course, many other reasons for failure to retrieve a memory (e.g., anatomical changes, coding changes, associative interference, state-dependent learning).

One is very personal about one's own personal reality. Meaning, value, and significance are attributed to different aspects of the reality. Explanations and justifications are generated to account for specifics of the reality. And one becomes attached, in varying degrees, to the perceptions, memories, thoughts, and beliefs.

REALIZING

In Conjunctive Psychology, therapies specifically aimed at altering the personal reality are called "realizing." Many of the practices logically follow from the above discussion of personal realities. For example, working with attachments, as discussed in the last chapter, is often a powerful realizing approach. Anorexics might be forced to look at photos of themselves to see what they really look like. Or discrimination training may produce necessary changes in schemas/categories, attributions, or beliefs. A person who holds that "All men . . . " or "The boss always . . . " may profit from discrimination learning. In assertiveness training, a client learns to discriminate an appropriately assertive behavior from one that is nonassertive or aggressive.

One of the most applicable and powerful realizing approaches is the cultivation of positive thinking. This is the most common and a very useful component in the vast self-help literature (e.g., Carnegie, 1948; Kaufman, 1977). It involves seeing reality from a positive orientation—seeing the glass half-full rather than half-empty—and thinking about life in terms of challenges and opportunities rather than obstacles. It does not involve distorting perception or deluding oneself so that reality seems more positive! This would be contrary to our mindfulness theme and to effective living. Rather, one wants to perceive and think accurately, but with a positive orientation. Using cognitive therapies and working with behaviors of the mind can help the client have more control over his thoughts and replace negative thoughts with positive ones. The second part of the Buddhist eightfold path is "right thought," which includes reducing lust, ill-will, and cruelty in thoughts.

Changing the words clients use to think about and describe their realities may facilitate discrimination learning, positive thinking, and other changes in the personal reality. For example, Vaughan (1995) recommends changing "shoulds" to "coulds" as a way of changing perception and thinking. "I should be more loving" becomes "I could be more loving, and I have a choice." While doing this, Vaughan recommends being mindful of any tendency to be judgmental or feeling discouraged. Enright (1996) suggests a "renaming" practice in which symptoms are renamed in order to see the situation in a more positive light. This helps clients see how the meaning and value one assigns to events affect how they are perceived and experienced. For one individual "stubborn" might be renamed "persistent." For another individual, "laziness" might be renamed "taking an unauthorized but well-deserved break."

Opportunities for realizing may occur when previously unconscious material emerges into consciousness. This might happen naturally as a result of encountering reminder stimuli, bodywork, dreams, drugs, meditation, or vision quests. It might result from psychoanalytic therapy that encourages exploration of the unconscious. This requires very skillful work by the helper. The rate of discovery has to be appropriate to the client; and as things are discovered, the helper must help the client understand, accept, and incorporate them (e.g., Shapiro et al., 1992). Behavior modification helps the client learn new ways of responding to some of the material.

An important part of the realizing therapies is for clients to come to understand and respect individual differences in personal realities. Such differences can be particularly dramatic across cultures (Lillard, 1998; Markus & Kitayama, 1991). There is not one "right" reality. For example, in marriage counseling, it may be useful for the clients to share their perceptions and try to see from the other's point of view, rather than argue about who was right. A good example of sharing different perceptions can be found in one use of the medicine wheel by the plains people of the Native Americans (Storm, 1972). The medicine wheel provides a structure that encourages the understanding that there are many different ways to perceive an object or idea (Freesoul, 1986). People may sit in a circle about the wheel at different points of view. An Indian's shield may illustrate some of his particular approaches, skills, goals, and guides (McGaa, 1990). Personal growth then involves learning from different ways of seeing as when traveling the wheel (Bear et al., 1991).

Various rites of passage, such as the Native American vision quest (Foster & Little, 1992), can be powerful vehicles of personal growth and changes in personal reality. There are changes in values and perceptions as one stage of a person's life dies and she is reborn into the next stage.

Most forms of psychological assessment have the potential to illuminate aspects of the client's personal reality. Writing and/or telling her personal story to the helper or the group can be revealing. For some clients, such as some children, nonverbal approaches may work better. The client can depict aspects of the personal reality via drawing, sculpting, dancing, or playing with given objects.

Although the term "mandala" can be described more specifically, as in Tibetan Buddhism, here it means a pictorial representation of aspects of one's personal reality. The client creates the mandala on a large piece of paper using something like felt pens, crayons, or paint, with a large choice of colors. He can also add photos, newspaper clippings, pins, stickers, etc. The mandala is filled with words, symbols, and pictures meaningful to the client. A person or personality trait might be represented by a simple figure. An emotion or force might be shown as an abstract splash of color. A sample of what might be in a mandala includes goals and aspirations, barriers and obstacles, attachments, emotions, mental factors, aspects of the self, friends and lovers, helpers and teachers, and transpersonal and cosmic forces. In addition to assessment uses, clients creating their own mandalas reflect more on their personal realities. The mandalas then can be good objects of meditation. Creating mandalas and contemplating one's own mandalas and other mandalas can be a useful part of personal and transpersonal growth and healing (Cornell, 1994; Fincher, 1991; Jung, 1959).

MYTHS AND STORIES

Myths and stories are a major way a culture shapes the personal realities of its members. Primarily influenced by mythologist Joseph Campbell, Western psychologists in the 1980s rediscovered the role of myths (Campbell & Moyers, 1988). This had a small impact on NAMAP and was a major cause for rekindled interest in Jung's psychology, which gives great weight to myths and symbols (Jung, 1964).

Myths help one to make sense of the world and assign meaning to aspects of one's personal reality, needs emphasized by developmental and existential theorists. Myths provide commonalties with others in the culture and are often acted out in rituals. Campbell suggested that myths serve four functions (Campbell, 1972; Campbell & Moyers, 1988). First is the mystical function, opening the world to the dimension of mystery. Second is the cosmological function, showing the nature of the universe in a way the mystery comes through. Third is the sociological function, supporting and validating the social order. And fourth is the pedagogical function, showing how to live a human life under any circumstances.

The integrative helper will be concerned when a client's personal mythology is dysfunctional and/or no longer satisfying. Perhaps the client has outgrown myths that served well in an earlier developmental stage. Perhaps the myths were shattered by a trauma. Perhaps the culture has changed in ways that make the myths less useful. Perhaps the myths have always been problematical or evil, such as encouraging aggression. In such cases, the helper may help clients become more aware of their myths and develop more functional and satisfying personal mythologies (Feinstein & Krippner, 1988; Keen & Valley-Fox, 1989). There are many practices that could be utilized here, such as reading stories, writing stories, journal work, guided fantasies, meditation, dream work, shamanic journeys, vision quests, spiritual reading and practices, art therapy, Gestalt therapy, and Jung's analytical psychotherapy.

Drawing from the world's myths, there are many images and concepts that can be useful in creating personal and communal mythologies, making mandalas, and conceptualizing treatment programs. For example, the idea of a warrior, which has been important to Native Americans and Tibetan Buddhists, has proven useful in parts of the American men's movement and treatment programs for aggressive teenagers. Other figures that can be approached mythically include Great Mother, Great Father, Queen, King, hero, expert, wiseperson, fool, lover, seducer, hunter, magician, artist, mystic, inner child, creator, destroyer, and observer.

Throughout history and all around the world, stories have been a major way cultures perpetuate themselves and pass on myths. Stories speak of many aspects of the human condition and experiences, and thus can be useful in personal growth. Stories can encourage people to reflect on and understand their situation. Sometimes, stories speak to people on a deeper or more symbolic level. People interested in women's issues, for example, may profit from stories about the psychological and spiritual nature of women (Estes, 1992) and/or stories of strong and heroic women (Phelps, 1981).

Clinically, in the field of bibliotherapy the client reads a story or has it read to him or her for the purpose of alleviating a psychological problem (Brown, 1975; Rubin, 1978). A child about to be hospitalized might be read a story about a child going to a hospital, explaining what will be encountered. Almost all bibliotherapy relies on understanding, insight, and/or attitude change to produce behavior change, such as reducing fears. But, as discussed earlier, such approaches have limited effectiveness with strong behaviors, such as strong fears. Hence, a relatively unexplored area of great potential is the incorporation of behavior modification procedures into stories, especially for children (Mikulas & Coffman, 1989; Mikulas et al., 1985).

Particularly powerful are teaching stories for personal/transpersonal growth (Feldman & Kornfield, 1991). Zen Buddhism (Reps, 1957) and the Sufis (Shah, 1971a), among others, are noted for their skillful use of such stories. Many of these stories, including Jesus' parables and Native American animal stories, can be understood at several different levels. Indries Shah (1971b) tells the Sufi story of Saadi's visit to the burial place of John the Baptist in Syria. He arrived exhausted and footsore. While feeling sorry for himself, he saw a man who was not only tired, but also had no feet. Saadi then gave thanks that at least he had feet. At one level, the moral of the story is to be thankful for what you have, a form of positive thinking. At a deeper level is the question, why does one have to see someone with no feet to appreciate having feet, or even to realize one has feet? Shah asks, "How much of my life is being wasted while I wait for someone to tell me what to do, or something to happen which will change my condition and frame of mind?"

PERSONAL REALITY EMERGENCY

Occasionally, there may be a relatively sudden and dramatic change in one's personal reality. This might include things such as unusual experiences and perceptions, challenges to one's values or sense of self, confrontation with repressed memories or parts of the self (perhaps symbolically or mythically, such as a fight with a demon), intense emotions, various fears, physical symptoms, indecision and inability to act, the arising of strange energies or apparent psychic powers, feelings of being overwhelmed, or exaggerations of the sense of self (e.g., "ego-inflation"). There are many possible causes for such a personal reality emergency, including stress, lack of sleep, significant life changes, personal trauma, near-death experience, drugs, disease, rising of kundalini, intense meditation, some spiritual practices, and psychotherapy.

Consider a client who is involved in a very unpleasant psychological process in which his basic sense of self and reality is being torn apart, and he is subjectively battling powerful demons. What should the helper do? In some cases, it is best to stop the process, as with drugs and/or institutionalization, because the process will hurt the client too much. This would be NAMAP's basic approach, usually calling it psychosis. But in other cases, it is best to allow and perhaps facilitate the process, because it leads to changes that the client later says made the process one of the most important and valuable events of his life. Many great artists, scientists, and mystics would have lost something important if they had been drugged as soon as things seemed somewhat "crazy."

Christina and Stanislav Grof (1989), who were primary instigators in the treatment of this type of case in the United States, termed such a situation a "spiritual emergency." They recognized that for some people this emergency can have a powerful positive outcome. The emergency can lead to a personal growth or healing experience, the next stage in development, and/or a greater integration of being. Sometimes, it leads to being "reborn," as described in many myths.

A critical question for integrative helpers is when to stop the process and when to allow it to continue. The Grofs (1990) suggest some criteria for when one may profit from the process: The experience is not due to a medical condition, the person is aware the process is related to spiritual/transpersonal issues, and the person is able to differentiate his inner experiences from the world of consensus reality. Lukoff (1985) described mystical experiences, psychotic episodes, and situations where they overlap. He suggested four criteria for the likelihood of positive outcomes from psychotic episodes: good pre-episode functioning; acute onset of symptoms during a period of three months or less; stressful precipitants to the psychotic episode, such as major life changes; and a positive exploratory attitude toward the experience as meaningful, revelatory, and growthful. Lukoff suggests that at least two of the four criteria must be present for a positive outcome.

If the process is allowed to continue, there are many ways the helper can facilitate it (Bragdon, 1990; Cortright, 1997; Grof & Grof, 1989, 1990; Stallone & Migdal, 1991). The helper aids the client in understanding what is happening in terms of the dynamics of the personal and transpersonal levels of being, using a conceptualization that speaks to the client, which may or may not be spiritual. With compassion and acceptance, the helper actively values the process to the client as meaningful and important, relieves the client of fears of going crazy, emphasizes that the emergency will pass, delineates possible negative and positive aspects of the process, and encourages a positive and productive attitude to the process. The helper assists the client in finding a safe and secure place for the process to unfold, a place where she will not be disturbed, not disturb others, and ideally be close to nature. In this place, the client needs the helper or an experienced guide to monitor and facilitate the work.

The helper encourages the client to express herself in various ways, such as verbally and via art, and allows for the common venting of emotions. It is often useful to help the client become more grounded through her body, as with movement, exercise, physical work, or mindfulness of body. The process can be slowed down through medication and nutrition. The client might be advised to eat foods such as grains, beans, dairy products, and perhaps meat, and avoid sugar and caffeine. During and after the process, the helper aids the client in incorporating the new experiences and insights, perhaps with the use of mandalas. Following the emergency, the helper helps the client with the transformation of the personal reality and integration back into daily living.

ALTERNATIVE PERSONAL REALITIES

Another way one's personal reality may dramatically change is through a change in state of consciousness, which may or may not be associated with an emergency. The dream state is the best example. The principles of reality of the dream state are very different from those of the waking state. The setting may instantly and dramatically change; one may be able to fly or change shape; another person may change into an animal. Such things are easy and not problematical in the dream state. Because the dream state reality is so different from the waking state reality, it is usually considered an example of an altered or different "state of consciousness" (Tart, 1975; Wolman & Ullman, 1986). But if consciousness is a field, it is not clear what a state of consciousness is. Hence, a more accurate term might be "state of being," "domain of consciousness," or "alternative personal reality." But for clarity of the present discussion, the accepted expression "state of consciousness" will be used.

Metzner (1989) defined a different state of consciousness as a time-limited state in which the patterns of thought, feeling or mood, and perception and sensation are altered from the ordinary or baseline condition. This includes changes in the sense of self. A different state of consciousness might result from drugs, disease, sensory overload, sensory complexity deprivation, meditation, pranayana, sacred dance, ritualistic magic, and occasionally hypnosis. In the United States, interest in different states grew dramatically during the 1960s due to greater use of mind-altering drugs, the influx of Eastern psychologies and spiritualities with maps and descriptions of different states, and the increased availability of meditators for research.

In a classic paper, Charles Tart (1972) pointed out that the laws of one state of consciousness do not necessarily apply to another state. Thus, it would be difficult, if not impossible, to adequately "understand" or "explain" the nature of one state of consciousness from the perspective of a different state. This results in what Tart calls a "state-specific science," a science based on one particular state. The trap for NAMAP and others is to take the science of the ordinary, awake, consensus state of consciousness, and apply it inappropriately to other states. Rather, we need to develop sciences specific to these other states. Theorists are gradually identifying concepts and dimensions for use in mapping and categorizing different states (e.g., Clark, 1983; Fisher, 1971; Ring, 1976; Walsh, 1995). Buddhism includes many mandalas with representations of different states of consciousness, such as the popular Wheel of Existence (cf. Metzner, 1996).

Andrew Weil (1973), among many others, argues that a drive to alter one's consciousness is a pervasive and natural feature of human consciousness. Children alter their consciousness by spinning and hanging upside down. Almost all known world cultures use some mind-altering substance, such as alcohol. Also around the world, altered states of consciousness, in client and/or practitioner, are a major way to facilitate healing and cultivate mental health (Grof, 2000; Ward, 1989). For example, to help heal a client, a shaman must be able to move back and forth between an ordinary state of consciousness and a shamanic state (Harner, 1980).

The important thing for the integrative helper to understand is that it is usually possible for one to learn how to move within and between states of consciousness. For example, rather than being impaired by some drug, such as marijuana, one can learn to actively explore the drug-induced state, gradually becoming more competent in that state. Then one can learn to move between the drug state and the normal state, eventually phasing out the need for the drug. However, this would seldom be the primary treatment of choice for drug problems. Similarly, in early stages of meditation practice, there is a distinct difference between when one is in a meditative state and when not. But as practice continues, this distinction diminishes. One learns how to cultivate a meditative stance in daily living.

Usually when one is dreaming, one is lost in that state, unaware that it is a dream. But it is possible for one to bring a waking type of awareness into the dream, known in the West as "lucid dreaming" (LaBerge, 1985). Here, one is aware that one is dreaming and one can explore and profit from the dream state. For example, one may seek out the wisdom of a particular dream figure. There are many ways to cultivate lucid dreaming (LaBerge & Rheingold, 1990). While awake you may regularly ask yourself whether you are is dreaming. This mental habit may carry over into the dream state. When the answer to the question is "yes" or "perhaps," try to do something that would be impossible in the waking state, such as fly. All this may produce lucid dreaming. Waking up in the dream state is an important Tibetan practice, known as dream yoga (Norbu, 1992; Wangyal, 1998). The purpose is to facilitate waking up from the normal waking state, moving into a transpersonal domain of consciousness.

It may be useful to think of some clients, perhaps classified as psychotic or schizophrenic, as being in an altered state of consciousness (Laing, 1960;

Lukoff, 1996; Ruitenbeek, 1972). Treatment should not consist of trying to force the person into consensus reality. Rather, the client should be helped and guided on a journey of inner space so as not to be overcome by experiences, but to profit from them. Then the person is gradually guided into consensus reality in a way that facilitates the integration of the different states.

To be most effective, it is usually best if the guide has had personal experience with the conscious domains the client is exploring or struggling with. A person who has worked his way out of a "schizophrenic" domain may be a good guide for another person similarly lost. To be a psychoanalyst, one must first go through psychoanalysis. To be a meditation teacher, one should have done a lot of meditating, not just read about it. And to help a person on a psychedelic voyage, it is useful if one has had similar experiences.

Finally, it should be stressed that one's beliefs have a strong effect on the availability and specifics of various states. After exploring different states of consciousness in a variety of ways, John Lilly (1972) concluded: "In the province of the mind, what is believed to be true is true or becomes true, within limits to be found experientially and experimentally. These limits are further beliefs to be transcended."

INTERACTIONS WITH OTHER LEVELS

Variables of the personal level naturally influence the biological level. Positive thinking promotes biological health. For example, Scheier and Carver (1987) report that realistic optimism improves cardiovascular responses, muscle enzyme activity, and immune system functioning. Part of this is because optimists are better at developing plans of action to solve problems (Scheier et al., 1986). In potential stress situations, a person's perceptions of, interpretations of, and attitudes toward events influence how much stress he will experience at the biological level (Pelletier, 1977; Sapolsky, 1998). And positive emotions often promote healthy perceptions, beliefs, and overall physical well-being (Salovey et al., 2000).

It is very important that the integrative helper never underestimate the great power of beliefs! This power can be seen in a wide variety of interrelated literatures including expectancy, placebo, psychosomatic, faith, and hypnosis (e.g., Harrington, 1997; Roberts et al., 1993; Wadden & Anderton, 1982; White et al., 1985). Placebo drugs and placebo psychological therapies often are significantly more effective than no treatment. Warts, which are probably due to a virus, are healed by a wide range of folk remedies based on the person's believing in the treatment. Many people have had major operations without pain, due only to hypnotic suggestion. And some people have died because of their belief in a curse put on them. In weight lifting, prior to 1970, no one had ever lifted 500 pounds over his head. Many argued it was a physiological impossibility. But in the month after Vasily Alexeev broke the barrier, four other weight lifters also lifted more than 500 pounds.

Many actions at the behavioral level are in response to perceptions, as manifested at the personal level, rather than to sensations at the biological level. That is, people often respond to their perceptions of the situations, rather than to the actual situations. This is a basis of the realizing therapies. Also, many behaviors are guided by the values and goals of the personal level. For example, people strive to achieve what they believe is important. Changes in values and goals may produce changes at the behavioral level by changes in what is reinforcing.

A major part of an individual's personal reality consists of justifications and explanations of behavior. This is what is really happening here and why it is good I did that. Also, the self may believe it was the agent of a behavior, when this is often a post hoc illusion. Delgado (1969) describes a patient who was forced to turn his head by electrical stimulation of the internal capsule of the brain. Although the stimulation produced simple movement, the patient explained the behavior: "I am looking for my slippers," "I heard a noise," and "I was looking under the bed." A famous American learning theorist was operantly shaped, without his awareness, to give his lectures while standing next to the side wall with windows. Reinforcement was based on students' subtle and differential attention, nodding, smiling, asking questions, and taking notes. When later asked why he stood at that wall, he honestly answered it was because he could see the blackboard better, due to reduced glare from the windows. (A reversal design showed the professor's explanation to be unlikely; he was conditioned to the wall, then away from the wall, then back to the wall.) Speaking from a yogic perspective, Jean Klein (1988, p. 63) described the mind in its normal state as "a restless, self-centered instrument rationalizing and justifying mechanical behaviour."

Helping clients become more mindful of their excuses and justifications can often help reduce obstacles to change and decrease the chance of relapse. For example, for the client who has recently quit smoking or drinking, it may be helpful to know in advance the most likely excuses to resume. Then when one of these excuses arises, it is a discriminative stimulus to stay mindful and not unconsciously give in, resist with an act of will, and perhaps employ a behavioral self-control technique. Typical excuses include "Just one won't hurt," "I can always stop again," "Right now I really need it," and "I currently have greater problems."

A common phenomenon, which occurs in many forms, is the "self-fulfilling prophecy" (Jones, 1986; Jussim, 1986). This refers to situations where people's beliefs and assumptions cause them to perceive and act in ways that result in events that confirm their beliefs. It often includes influencing other people to act in expected ways. This has been shown many times in classrooms, where teachers' expectations about students may produce behavior in the students that matches what the teachers expect (Jussim, 1986; Rosenthal & Jacobson, 1968). Consider Ann and Bonny, two children who are equally smart and creative. The teacher, however, believes Ann is much sharper than Bonny. When answering a question, Ann gives a somewhat unusual answer, which the teacher perceives as creative; thus, she rewards Ann. When Bonny gives a somewhat unusual answer, the teacher perceives it as a stupid error and punishes Bonny. As a result of such dynamics, Ann does better in school, is more motivated, and enjoys it more, as the teacher could have predicted.

The self-fulfilling prophecy is one of the problems with putting psychological/psychiatric labels on people (Szasz, 1970). People may respond to the person on the basis of the label and influence the person to act in ways that fit the label. Relatedly, the labeled person may tend to act in ways that fit his beliefs about how such a person acts.

The integrative helper needs to be alert for self-fulfilling prophecies that have caught the client. For example, Susan believed that people would not accept her because of her appearance and lifestyle. As a result, she had few friends and did not fit well into the community. In fact, her beliefs were largely groundless. But because of her beliefs, she misperceived other people, which led her to act in ways that caused others to be more reserved and less friendly, which caused Susan. . . . Susan had the behavioral skills, motivation, and values to be a good friend and valuable member of the community, but she needed realizing therapy to free her from the self-fulfilling prophecy.

The idea that through our beliefs we create our own reality is a common part of "new age" philosophy and the basis of some related personal/spiritual programs (e.g., est, Avatar). Although things are not as simple or magical as sometimes described and promised, we can see how the self-fulfilling prophecy can contribute, to some extent, in our creating our reality. Here are two more examples. A professional pickpocket in New York City was asked how he knew whom to rob and where their valuables were. He said that many people give it away, such as the man who periodically touches his jacket pocket where his wallet is, to be sure it is still there and safe. So people who are very concerned about being robbed may act in ways that make it more likely they will be robbed.

Consider two people, Rob who practices positive thinking and Al who focuses on the negative. Rob seeks out and is sought out by other positive-thinking people, and they all tend to avoid very negative people. Al, on the other hand, spends time with other negative people who share his complaints about the job, world, women. Rob lives in a much happier and more pleasant world than Al does.

Understanding the nature and relativity of one's personal reality is a necessary prerequisite for some types of personal growth. To the extent that people are attached to the specifics of their personal reality, they are impaired in trying to change that reality, as in discovering the transpersonal level of being. Moving into more expansive domains of consciousness generally requires people to recognize and release their hold on a more limited view. The yogic/vedantic term "maya" is usually translated "illusion," which in some yogic schools means something very like the personal reality. From this perspective, when yogic psychology talks about people living in illusion, it does not deny the relative reality and personal importance of the personal reality. But it affirms that there is something more, which is more "real" or more "absolute" in some sense. A common result of exploring many different states of consciousness is the sense of a more fundamental ground or domain in which the various states are special cases, plays, or dances.

In the transition from the personal to the transpersonal, there are developmental sequences to some states of consciousness. And one can talk about different levels of consciousness, where a higher level includes all of the lower level, but also contains more. For example, in the Buddhist/yogic literatures, there are detailed descriptions of different states and levels that result from intermediate and advanced practice of concentration and mindfulness meditation (Buddhaghosa, 1975; Goleman, 1988). These lead from the personal level to the transpersonal level.

This chapter has focused on the self-centered personal reality, with a number of references to the self. In the next chapter, this self will be examined more closely.

SUMMARY

The personal level is defined in terms of a conscious personal reality inhabited by a personal self that acts through the agency of will. The personal reality is a learned reality, influenced by the intermix of culture, language, and gender. It is unique to the individual and can be partially represented by a mandala. Clinically and interpersonally, it is often important for a person to come to understand and respect another person's reality.

Perceptions and memories in a personal reality are influenced by learning, motivation, and attachments. Such mental contents are often distorted in ways to make them fit more closely the assumptions and biases of the personal reality. This distortion can have a variety of psychological consequences.

Realizing therapies are ways to alter the personal reality. This includes discrimination learning, reducing attachments, positive thinking, and changing the words and myths used to describe and explain. Previously unconscious material that arises into consciousness may result in changes in the personal reality.

Sometimes there is a dramatic change in the personal reality, as in a personal reality emergency or an alternative personal reality. Most helpers will not encounter these (other than dreams); and if they do, they probably will not have the expertise or facilities to work with them. But the helper must realize that some people in a personal reality emergency can be guided through the emergency, coming out with a more integrated personality and/or a furthering of development. And some people having trouble with alternative personal realities can learn to move within and between different states of consciousness. The integrative helper refers such people to helpers who specialize in these areas.

AUTHOR'S REFLECTIONS

It is one thing to understand intellectually that one's personal reality is learned. It is another thing to have an existential realization of the significance of this fact. Such a realization makes it easier for people to change their personal realities and discover more basic domains of reality. As the esoteric Gurdjieff often said, to escape from prison a person must first realize that he is in prison.

Myths and stories can be a powerful part of education, personal growth, and clinical work. A story or metaphor is often remembered better and longer than other information. For example, in talks and workshops, I often describe in detail the drunken monkey. Years later, some people remember the monkey well, but little else of what was said. Integrative helpers collect stories that are useful with their population of clients.

The field of bibliotherapy, particularly with children, is wide open for new innovative research and applications. For example, the two references in the chapter is the total literature on building behavior modification into children's stories. There is great potential here. On a more general level, there is considerable opportunity to incorporate teaching stories and psychological instruction into books, plays, television programs, and other media. Perhaps some of you will be involved in this.

THOUGHT QUESTIONS

1. There are some advantages to the Vedanta position that consciousness is superordinate to individual brains, versus the position that consciousness is a product of brains. One is that it can explain telepathy more easily. How might telepathy work? What is another advantage to the Vedanta position?
2. Imagine in detail some very emotional event and observe the effects on your body. What did you observe? What are the implications of such effects?
3. Give a detailed example of how race or gender affects one person's perceptions.
4. For a hypothetical case, describe how a therapist unintentionally implants a false memory in a client.
(5.) List two examples of how your past has influenced the way in which you construct your personal reality.
(6.) What areas of your personal reality are "not open for discussion?"
(7.) Give examples of how changing your personal reality or personal myth would help reduce negative behaviors or emotions you currently engage in or experience.
8. How does reducing attachments work as a realizing therapy?
9. How could you use a variation of the medicine wheel in group therapy?
10. Describe the specific use of a mandala with a hypothetical client.
11. Create your own personal tarot deck, using some of the cards from a regular deck. The suit of hearts is concerned with love and personal relationships; spades, with concerns and problems; diamonds, with vocation and hobbies; clubs, with personality. (You can, of course, assign different meanings to the suits.) For individual cards, write on them specific issues, attributes, or characteristics related to that suit in your life. Describe how you would use such a personal tarot (e.g., contemplation, meditation, seeing new relationships, breaking set). Be specific.
12. Give examples of how your personal myths fulfill the four functions described by Campbell.
13. Give an example of a teaching story that is significant to you.
(14.) How do myths and stories affect cultures?

15. Give an example of a myth that a person has outgrown and a myth that is dysfunctional.
16. Describe a hypothetical case of a personal reality emergency and how it leads to a greater integration of being.
(17.) In what ways might an altered state of consciousness be used to aid in treating a woman who has been raped?
(18.) Think for a moment about how your beliefs and schemas have impacted the ways in which you have interpreted the material in this chapter. How might your interpretation differ if you had spent much of yesterday in very different states of consciousness?
(19.) Give an example in your life of a self-fulfilling prophecy.
(20.) With our knowledge of self-fulfilling prophecies, how must we be cautious in therapy?
21. How do changes at the personal level result in changes at the biological and behavioral levels?

SELF AND WILL

The self is the center of the personal reality. From the self's perspective, the self is a conscious entity that is the observer of the perceptions and the willful agent responsible for many behaviors. The self is the central star in the great melodrama of the personal reality. Much of a person's happiness and suffering is based on the experiences, accomplishments, and adventures of the self in the melodrama.

The self is best understood by experiential knowing, supported by conceptual knowing. Therefore, the next section is devoted to facilitating and eliciting experiential knowledge of one's self. Readers are very strongly encouraged to give serious attention to the questions and allow sufficient time to reflect on and answer them. The best way is to take one paragraph at a time, in order, ideally not reading ahead. There are no "right" or "wrong" answers, only what is true for the reader. Also, a question may not yield any answer. Most people profit by writing down their answers. Over time, you should be mindful of how the answers change.

QUESTIONS AND SELF-MEDITATIONS

Who am I? What is your best answer or answers to this classic question about yourself? How would you define or describe your self? What is your personal first-hand experience of this self?

What are my attitudes and feelings, positive and negative, toward my self? How do you feel about your self? What do you like and dislike? How would some of these feelings be represented in a mandala (a pictorial representation of part of one's reality)? What would be the form, color, and content of these representations?

Where am I? Where does this self live? What is your firsthand experience of the location of the self? Almost everyone falls into one or more of the following categories: I am inside my head, looking out through my eyes, with a body below. I am inside the middle of my body, perhaps in the heart or hara (Japanese: "underbody" or "belly"; Zen: spiritual center). I completely fill up my body, extending out into all fingers, toes, and so on. I exist outside of my body, such as at a place behind and above my head.

How do I experience my self as the observer? What is your firsthand experience of the observer? For example, when visual perception is occurring, there is the object of the perception, the process of seeing, and the self as observer. What is your experience of the observer self, and can you separate this experience from the experience of the object and perhaps the experience of seeing? This is very difficult.

How do I experience my self as the actor? Willfully and slowly do some simple action, such as move a finger. What is your direct experience of the agent who wills the action? What is your experience of the process of willing? Again, difficult questions.

Do I shift between a number of distinctively different selves? These different selves might arise in different personal or professional roles, or when in different situations or with different people. For example, one woman might have a tough, logical, business self; a consistent, concerned, loving, mother self; an impulsive, sensitive, lover self; and a fragile, vulnerable, child self. How would you represent your different selves in a mandala?

NATURE OF THE SELF

Western psychology includes massive literatures related to the self (e.g., Brinthaupt & Lipka, 1992; Hoyle et al., 1999; Lapsley & Power, 1988; Segal & Blatt, 1993; Suls, 1982; Suls & Greenwald, 1983, 1986; Wright, 1977). There is no need to survey or review these literatures here. Rather, emphasis will be given to a few points important to the integrative helper and themes of this book.

In these literatures, there are a number of related terms: self, ego, self-identity, personal identity, and soul. There is no consensus in how these terms are used, both among and within different schools of thought. For example, within various psychoanalytic theories, there is little agreement on what is meant by "self." And across clinical and personality theories, sometimes "self" and "ego" mean basically the same thing, and sometimes they are significantly different. The first paragraph of this chapter gives the Conjunctive Psychology description of the self. The self is the conscious center of the personal reality, a seeming observer of perceptions and willful agent of some behaviors. This approach to the self is compatible with all the Eastern psychologies. In some yogic and Hindu cosmologies, a distinction is emphasized between the ego or self at the personal level and a transcendental Self at the transpersonal level.

An important distinction is between the self as subject and the self as object, what William James (1890) called the I versus me. The self as object includes the various thoughts, memories, and feelings one has toward one's self, as reflected in the answers to the first two questions of the preceding section. The self as subject includes the experiences of one's self as observer and actor, as in the answers to questions four and five. The self as object cuts across the first three levels of being: body; behaviors, including social and professional roles; personal melodrama. The self as subject arises in the personal level and provides a gate to the transpersonal level, as discussed in the next chapter.

Because the self is part of the personal reality, all of the dynamics described in the last chapter apply to the self! For example, perceptions and memories are altered and constructed to fit one's beliefs and attachments related to one's self. And something that is too challenging to one's image of one's self will not be allowed into consciousness unaltered (Curtis, 1992). Greenwald (1980) discussed three self-based cognitive biases: egocentricity, where the self is perceived as more central to events than it really is; "beneffectance," where the self is selectively perceived as responsible for desired, but not undesired, outcomes; and conservation, resistance to cognitive change.

In some cases, self-based distortions and illusions may enhance self-esteem, maintain beliefs in personal efficacy, and promote an optimistic view of the future; these then may promote the ability to care about others, the ability to engage in productive and creative work, and the ability to be happy and content (Taylor & Brown, 1988). On the other hand, self-caused distortions and illusions often result in many psychological problems and personal suffering. Such cases may require a realizing therapy (previous chapter) or a self therapy (below).

An extremely important dynamic of the self is self-perpetuation, active maintenance of the sense of self and construction of a sense of a continual self across time (e.g., Andrews, 1991). The memory system is enslaved by the self for this purpose. Memories are constructed to include the self and/or to center on the self, as a way to create the illusion of a constant historical self. Similarly with fantasies of the future. And most religions thrive on promises of eternal existence for some variation of the self or soul.

Quite extraordinary is the tendency for a person to behave continually in maladaptive ways, because it perpetuates some attached view of the self. A person will continually make the same errors in perception, thought, and/or action, even though these errors continually cause problems and suffering. The great inertia to change results from the person's being attached to a sense of self that has such perceptions, thoughts, and actions. Perhaps the person is more comfortable with the known self, even with its problems, than with the idea of some new or different self. Perhaps the person has personally and/or professionally committed his self to certain views and opinions; and to change would require acknowledging being "wrong," which is a problem for many people. Integrative helpers need to be alert to this type of self-based inertia, because it is very common and can be very influential. "For example, people with negative self-views seek relationship partners who view them negatively, elicit unfavorable evaluations from partners, and 'see' more negativity in the reactions of others than is actually there" (Swann, 1997, p. 177). Here the motive to verify and maintain a particular view of the self overrides the disadvantages of the self-fulfilling prophecy.

CROSS-CULTURAL INFLUENCES

The culture has a strong influence on the development and nature of the self, thus creating significant cross-cultural differences (Geertz, 1973; Landrine, 1992; Markus & Kitayama, 1991; Rothbaum et al., 2000). One of the best-known and most important distinctions is between the independent self and the interdependent self, referred to as the independent self-construal versus the interdependent self-construal (Markus & Kitayama, 1991) and the referential self versus the indexical self (Landrine, 1992). A third alternative of no self, which may exist in some cultures (Landrine, 1992), will be discussed in the next chapter.

The independent self is a unique, bounded, autonomous entity that is distinct and separate from other selves. The American cowboy is a typical mythical symbol. The interdependent self, on the other hand, is constituted, defined, and influenced by social roles, relationships with significant others, cultural contexts, and group harmony. The interdependent self thus includes other people and parts of the world, which are clearly "non-self" to the independent self. The interdependent self is dominant in East Asia and can be found in many American minorities. Western white men have primarily independent selves, while women are more interdependent (Cross & Madson, 1997).

Western psychology and NAMAP have been dominated by theories of development, personality, mental health, and morality, which were promoted by white males and glorify the independent self. This has, of course, created numerous practical, social, and ethical problems related to psychological assessment and treatment. For example, women with interdependent selves have often gotten poorer assessments of mental health and/or morality than if they had independent selves. Western psychotherapeutic goals of self-integration and self-actualization would be condemned in traditional Arabic societies that value the collective identity over the independent self (Dwairy & Van Sickle, 1996). On the other hand, from the perspective of a Western psychology based on the independent self, the interdependent self is an example of psychopathology (e.g., failure to maintain ego boundaries) (Landrine, 1992).

Thus, the integrative helper needs to assess and take into account where the client is on the continuum from independent to interdependent. For example, with a client with a more interdependent self, the family might be more involved in the therapy and more attention may be given to helping the client fulfill or change social roles (Landrine, 1992). The independent client may be more motivated by anger, frustration, and pride; while the interdependent client may be more motivated by indebtedness, empathy, and shame (Markus & Kitayama, 1991). And some of the strategies in this book, such as the self-control emphasis, may need to be approached differently with the interdependent client than with the dependent client (e.g., Rothbaum et al., 2000; Weisz et al., 1984).

Of course, each client is unique and there are many ways that culture and other experiences can influence the nature of the self. The integrative helper learns about the client's culture and how it might impact therapy issues and approaches. But most important are the client's beliefs, attitudes, thoughts, and perceptions related to the personal self. These might be revealed with variations of the questions asked earlier.

SELF THERAPIES

There are at least five, overlapping therapeutic approaches that focus on the self. The approaches emphasize self as object, integration of self, self-related attachments, transcendence of self, and restructuring the self.

The self as object approach, discussed below, deals with the thoughts, feelings, and attitudes one has toward one's self. These are important in an absolute sense, but also how they compare to some standard, goal, or ideal imposed by self and/or others. The self as object is the source of many personal-level problems and a main focus of the humanistic therapies.

Integration of the self involves two, often overlapping, approaches. First, is integration of previously unconscious material that has naturally arisen for reasons listed in the last chapter (e.g., dreams, drugs, bodywork) and/or is intentionally sought through psychoanalysis (e.g., Freud, Jung). Ideally, the client integrates this material into a new, broader, enriched, personal reality. Jung includes integrating in the "shadow," the dark, feared, and unwanted aspects of one's being (Zweig & Abrams, 1990). Jung felt this would lead to greater self-acceptance, new potentials, and healing relationships with others. The second type of integration of self involves the integration of multiple selves or subpersonalities, as discussed below.

The third self therapy, discussed below, focuses on attachments related to the self. This includes how attachments produce distortions in thought and perception, self-fulfilling prophecies, and resistance to change.

The fourth self therapy, discussed in the next chapter, involves gradual transcendence of the self. One disidentifies with the self of the personal level and thus escapes some of the unnecessary suffering of the personal melodrama. Transcendence of the self would very rarely be the sole form of self therapy, although it is always possible for anyone. However, the integrative helper often works on several levels simultaneously. Thus, adding a transcendence component to another form of self therapy, particularly attachment work, can be very powerful. Otherwise, one can get indefinitely lost doing repair work on various aspects of self and personality. As a vehicle of self-perpetuation, the self loves self-work and will continually create related melodramas (e.g., Now I am in therapy. Now I am doing spiritual work. Look, it's me on another adventure!).

The fifth form of self therapy involves restructuring the self. Here the psychoanalyst helps the client reform the self or ego so that it is more stable, cohesive, and purposive, and is better at adaptation, growth, and interfacing with the world. During the 20th century CE, psychoanalysis moved from the drive-centered approach of Freud to a more self-centered approach that involves enhancing and restructuring the self (e.g., Kohut, 1971, 1977). This has brought psychoanalysis into closer conjunction with humanistic approaches, which emphasize the self (Kahn, 1985).

There is, however, a major problem in this approach: No psychoanalyst has ever found a self (or ego, or underlying cause). This is no surprise to the Buddhist psychologist, since a fundamental Buddhist principle of existence is that there is no separate, constant, entity of a self. One can easily find phenomena that can be interpreted as results of an assumed self; but the self as an entity remains elusive from direct perception and measurement. The Zen master might ask the client to show her this self that is of such concern.

A similar issue arises in contemporary Western cognitive therapies and social psychology. Here all of the dynamics of the self discussed above, such as selective attention, memory distortion, and self-perpetuation are often attributed to "self-schemas" (Markus, 1990; Stein & Markus, 1996). Therapy, personal growth, and behavior change then ultimately require change in such schemas. But, however heuristic the concept of self-schema proves to be, it is very unlikely that anyone will be able to actually find such a thing in a concrete sense.

Thus, in Conjunctive Psychology, no attempt is made to hunt down a self or self-schema. Rather, change procedures are employed that could be interpreted as producing changes in the self or self-schema. It is easy to make a level error here. For example, the fact that a client appears to have problems related to a self does not necessarily mean that the most effective form of therapy focuses on the personal level. Perhaps behavior modification is called for, which then produces changes in the self or self-schema.

SELF AS OBJECT

The self as object includes all the thoughts, memories, opinions, attitudes, and feelings one has toward one's self. It is revealed in the answers to the above questions "Who am I?" and "What are my attitudes and feelings, positive and negative, toward my self?" It includes the rich literatures about self-concept and self-esteem.

Self-concept includes the various thoughts and perceptions one has about one's self (Gergen, 1971; Hamachek, 1992; Lynch et al., 1981). Gecas and Mortimer (1987) suggest that self-concept encompasses the two dimensions of identity and self-evaluation. Identity has three aspects: role identity (e.g., father), character (e.g., honest), and existential identity (e.g., continuous). Self-evaluation also has three aspects: competence (e.g., feelings of efficacy), morality (e.g., feelings of self-esteem), and authenticity (e.g., sense of realness). Focusing on the self-concept is a central feature of humanistic therapy, particularly the "person-centered therapy" of Carl Rogers (1951, 1961).

The construct of self-esteem, which overlaps self-concept, includes a person's general attitudes and feelings toward one's self, such as how comfortable she is with herself and her feeling of self-worth (Bednar et al., 1989; Branden, 1969; Brockner, 1988). Rogers argued that the most important factor in self-esteem is being accepted and respected by significant others. Self-esteem depends on how a person experientially defines the self. If she defines her self in terms of social and professional roles, then self-esteem will depend on how "successful" she is in these roles. For another person, self-esteem may be based on living and acting according to chosen principles and beliefs.

Humanistic therapies for self as object help clients become more accepting of themselves and reduce conflicts within the self-concept. This includes building up positive aspects of self-concept and self-esteem and reducing negative aspects (Centi, 1981). Cognitive therapies and cognitive behavior therapy can change specific problematical cognitions that are part of self as object.

However, one of the most important facts of human psychology, and a significant part of Conjunctive Psychology, is the understanding that usually the best way to change self-concept and self-esteem is by changes at the behavioral and biological levels! Changes in self as object will usually result from such things as making the body healthier and more attractive, developing social and vocational skills, reducing unwanted emotions, forgiving others, and doing something you have wanted to do, such as take an art class or quit a job. Since we are observers of our behavior and our minds tend to justify our behavior, changes in behavior often lead to changes in our sense of self.

Many problems have arisen from not understanding these relationships. For example, some educators noted a correlation between students' poor academic skills and their low self-esteem. A number of long and costly programs were developed to enhance students' self-esteem as a way to improve their academic performance. This, of course, did not work. Trying to get students to generally feel better about themselves does not teach them how to study, how to take tests, how to think critically, how to use the computer, etc. On the other hand, if students are taught needed academic and social skills and, as a result, do better academically, their self-esteem will usually change to match.

There are, of course, many exceptions to the above discussion. For some clients, after biological and behavioral changes, there is still a need for a therapy aimed at the self as object. And there are some clients for whom the helper would begin with or emphasize a self therapy. How to assess these different types of situations is an area that requires more research and thought. Also, there are important cultural differences. For example, in North America the need for positive self-concept and self-esteem is often a powerful motivator; while in Japan a self-critical focus is more encouraged and appropriate (Heine et al., 1999).

A person not only develops and identifies with a sense of self, but will also compare this self with some standard, goal, ought self, or ideal self. This ideal self might be based on parents' teachings and examples, cultural socialization, television programming, social and vocational peer behavior, or spiritual commandments. The ideal self might be appropriate, ethical, or inspirational; or it might be inappropriate, problematical, or no longer useful. It is often important for the integrative helper to understand the nature of the ideal self.

Comparison of the self with the ideal self may help guide behavioral change and personal growth. One does things that change the self as object. Then one compares the self with the ideal self and continues doing the same types of things or moves in a new direction. This is a standard feedback system: behave, check results against goal, and adjust behavior appropriately. Stein and Markus (1996) suggest the idea of "possible selves," images of the self in the future that provide the cognitive foundation for goal-directed behavior.

The comparison of self and ideal self often produces a state of unsatisfactoriness, an important example of dukkha in Buddhist psychology. This dukkha often manifests as personal suffering and/or undesired affect, such as anxiety or depression (Higgins, 1987; Rogers, 1961). A young adult is not comfortable with a parent because she believes she is not the person expected or demanded by the parent. A person has a midlife crisis on his fiftieth birthday because he has not achieved everything his fantasy self contains, even though what he has achieved is more than ample for a happy, fulfilled life.

The negative affect from the comparison is a powerful motivator to do something to reduce the affect (Hamilton et al., 1993). What one does is reinforced by the decrease in negative affect (negative reinforcement), the basis of escape and avoidance conditioning. This might productively motivate the person toward desired goals. This is also a major way a culture influences its members to conform to social norms. An interdependent self might be particularly affected by shame and the desire to save face.

A person might act to avoid the dukkha from the self versus ideal self comparison. She might misperceive a situation or remember it differently so that there is less or no discrepancy. She might avoid making a decision, because a choice that turns out poorly could impact her view of herself as a competent decision maker (Larrick, 1993). Or she might engage in some behavior, such as binge eating, that pulls awareness away from the self versus ideal self comparison (Heatherton & Baumeister, 1991).

Therapies related to the self versus ideal self discrepancy change the ideal self, facilitate behavioral strategies to reduce the discrepancy, and/or reduce the dukkha caused by the discrepancy. If the ideal self is inappropriate, unreasonable, or undesirable, then a change in this standard may be necessary. A perfectly attractive teenage girl may feel she needs cosmetic surgery to make her look more like some currently trendy ideal. A college student may struggle with chemistry classes to be the doctor his parents want, when his heart is really in social work. A beginning meditator may quit the practice because he couldn't get his mind under control in the first three weeks.

If the ideal self is a reasonable and appropriate goal for the client, then the helper may help the client devise a plan of action to move in that direction. The key here is to break down the path to the ideal self into a series of reasonable and achievable minigoals. A person can be daunted by the long path, and so he needs to focus on the next step.

Finally is the issue of discrepancy-elicited dukkha and related negative affect. Although such affect may be a necessary and useful form of motivation in early and middle stages of development, eventually it is unnecessary and problematical. Getting free from this affect will be discussed in the next section and next chapter. A person makes friends with himself so that he is accepting of his current self, while simultaneously recognizing the value of change. He systematically works toward reasonable goals, with self-esteem based on making a good try, not on distance from some ideal self.

SELF-RELATED ATTACHMENTS

Working with attachments is a central part of yogic psychology and Conjunctive Psychology, and some of the most powerful attachments are related to the self. Self-perpetuation and resistance to change, discussed earlier, are accented when a person is attached to some self, even when the behaviors associated with this self are creating problems. The greater the attachment, the greater will be the need to protect, defend, perpetuate, and explain one's self. Thus, a person may explain his behavior to others, in an attempt to maintain some self-image. Or a person might continue an established role, such as being a witty person or sage, even when such behaviors are not appropriate. Attachments to the self often make the personal reality particularly self-centered. A person may say something in a small group and later have exaggerated beliefs about the others' thoughts concerning what was said. In fact, it may have had little or no impact and was forgotten by the others shortly thereafter.

As discussed in Chapter 7, attachments may cause distortion of perception, impairment in thinking, and undesired emotions. An individual will misperceive situations and alter memories of events in ways that will better fit his concept of himself. A person might perceive and remember himself as being charmingly clever at a social gathering, when, in fact, he was sarcastic and offensive. A person may lose some clarity and objectivity in thinking when the topic is threatening to him or suggests that the self needs to change. A person consuming too much alcohol may perceive himself as a moderate drinker with no serious alcohol-related problems. As a result, he does not adequately and clearly consider arguments to the contrary from friends and relatives.

The more attached you are to the self, the more likely you will experience negative affect when there are challenges to the self. Anxiety, anger, frustration, and depression are very common examples. One of these might occur when you perceive yourself behaving in ways that don't fit your self-image, or when social feedback suggests that you are different from the way you think you are. If a person is attached to a self-concept of being a compassionate person, and if someone points out behavior that is not compassionate, she will probably experience negative affect. If she were not attached, then she could use the feedback to become more compassionate. But the more attached she is, the less she can profit from the feedback, the more emotion will be elicited, and the more she will explain and rationalize the questionable behavior as really being compassionate. Consider the earlier discussion of comparing the self with the ideal self. Why should this be so emotional, as opposed to the more neutral guiding feedback some cognitive theorists suggest? The emotion is a sign of an attachment. Perhaps the person is attached to the idea that he should be the ideal self now, and/or he is attached to the current self, which resists change.

Ways to reduce attachments are discussed in Chapter 7. Included are attitude, awareness, and action. A person cultivates an attitude of taking delight in discovering attachments. This is coupled with mindfulness training to be more aware of the attachments and their precursors. Then he utilizes a plan of action to reduce the attachment, such as a behavioral self-control skill or a transpersonal transcendence practice.

Consider a parent responding to the misbehavior of a child. What is harmful to the child's self-concept and self-esteem is to convey to the child that he is a bad or unlovable person because of the behavior. Rather, the parent should convey to the child that she will always love the child unconditionally, but some behaviors are unacceptable. Similarly, with a good friend. The friend, like all people, will have positive and negative characteristics and behaviors, some of which are simply accepted and some of which you encourage the friend to change. But, ideally, you love the friend unconditionally regardless. This approach can be extended to cover everyone and is a powerful transpersonal practice. The point is to differentiate between the behavior of a person, which may be desirable or not, and the essence of a person, which is always lovable. Most people find this easier to do with others, such as a child, a friend, or a client, than with themselves.

All of this relates to important attachment and transcendence work. To the extent that a person's self is identified with his behaviors, there will be resistance to changing the behaviors and negative emotions when the behaviors do not match some ideal. So the integrative helper helps the client realize that he is not his behaviors. In addition, his true being is perfectly fine, even though many behaviors need to be changed. This is a powerful therapeutic strategy that facilitates behavior change, develops positive self-esteem, and encourages the transcendence process.

The same strategy applies to the contents of the mind. Most people are lost in the contents of their minds, which become their entire realities. Thus, the self becomes equated with some of the contents, self as object. Then the person becomes attached to some of the contents, self-related and other. This results in resistance to change, a problem for the client and helper. But the contents of the mind are just mental stuff, not who the person really is. As a result of meditation practice, a person may disidentify with the contents of the mind, perhaps identifying for awhile with the observer of the contents. This is often a very freeing experience for the meditator and raises the question, "If I am not the contents of my mind, which I used to believe, then who am I?" This disidentification reduces attachments to the contents, and thus greatly facilitates cognitive change.

MULTIPLE SELVES

For simplicity and clarity, the discussion so far has referred to a single self, but it is often useful to think about a person having several selves (e.g., Gergen, 1991). These different selves are sometimes called subpersonalities, self-schemas, or self-aspects. Different selves might be revealed by the earlier question, "Do I shift between a number of distinctively different selves?" Different situations and people may tend to elicit different selves. The memory system helps perpetuate each self and associate it with specific attributes and memories.

Sometimes the selves are in conflict with each other, creating problems for the person. In these cases, it is desirable to integrate the selves, as discussed below. A common psychoanalytic assumption is that the integration of all selves into one coherent structure is necessary for psychological health.

On the other hand, sometimes having multiple selves is advantageous to the person (Linville, 1987; Stein & Markus, 1994). For example, if one self fails, it does not mean all selves fail; a situation that elicits stress or anger in one self does not automatically impact the other selves. Self-concept and self-esteem can be very self-specific. Linville (1987) gives the following example: Ann has two basic selves, wife and lawyer, which are closely associated because her husband is also a lawyer with whom she has shared many professional experiences. When Ann gets divorced, the related negative affect and negative self-appraisal will be great because they spill over to affect her thoughts and feelings about both selves. In contrast, Dot has several, more distinct selves: wife with an electrician husband, lawyer, tennis player, and friend. Because the wife self is separate from the other selves, when Dot gets divorced, the negative aspects are less likely to spill over and affect her other selves. The other selves provide a buffer against the negative feelings associated with the divorce. Thus, therapy may help the client develop distinctions among different selves and focus on the positive, such as realizing that although one has marital problems one may still be a good parent (Linville, 1987). Discrimination learning, realizing therapy, and cognitive therapy may be applicable here.

The most extreme example of multiple selves is "multiple selves disorder," traditionally called "multiple personality disorder" and "dissociative identity disorder" (Beahrs, 1982; Braun, 1986). In multiple selves disorder, the person usually has many selves, often more than a dozen, some of which may not be aware of the others. A person may not be aware of being a multiple but is puzzled by blackouts or lost time that cannot be accounted for, new clothes in the closet never seen before, or phone calls from unknown lovers. The selves may differ in age, gender, speech, posture, values, and ideas. Multiples are predominantly female, highly suicidal, and with many somatic complaints. One self may not be aware of the suicidal self and cannot remember the suicide attempt that led to hospitalization.

Historically, multiple selves disorder was attributed to demonic or spirit possession. Now, it is generally believed that most cases began with sexual and/or physical abuse as a child. As a psychological defense, the self to which this happened is split off and compartmentalized, as a way of limiting the impact of the trauma. This primes the system to use the same strategy in other situations, and thus creates additional selves. For example, a self can be created that acts in ways that the main self would be embarrassed to do. Therapy for multiples has traditionally tried to integrate or "fuse" the various selves, usually with the aid of hypnosis (Beahrs, 1982; Braun, 1986).

As mentioned above, integration of selves is often helpful to people who don't have multiple selves disorder. This involves eliciting and/or fantasizing various selves; letting them express themselves in speech, writing, and/or art; and encouraging them to communicate with each other (e.g., Elliott & Greenberg, 1997). Sometimes the client is instructed to be mindful of these selves, cultivating an objective observer of the selves, while honoring and respecting the different points of view (e.g., Stone & Winkelman, 1989).

Emphasis on integration of selves is found in psychosynthesis, the personal growth approach developed by Roberto Assagioli (Assagioli, 1965; Whitmore, 1991). Assagioli suggested that there is a natural tendency for one to harmonize and synthesize various aspects of being at ever-higher levels of organization. Psychosynthesis is an attempt to cooperate with this tendency. It includes personal psychosynthesis, which involves the integration, control, and balancing of various selves, called "subpersonalities," around a personal-level self. This might be followed by transpersonal psychosynthesis, which involves integration around a transpersonal-level self. In personal psychosynthesis, the client is encouraged to confront his various subpersonalities, as through imagination or guided imagery. The subpersonalities are recognized, accepted, coordinated, and integrated. The main way this is done is by objectively observing the subpersonalities without identifying with them (mindfulness). According to Assagioli, this leads to a disidentification with the subpersonalities and the realization of a true personal self. This personal self may be given a mythical name, such as hero or artist, and is developed through visualization, imagery, and guided fantasy. As this self develops, the assumption is that it will be better able to integrate and control the subpersonalities.

Psychosynthesis contains a wide variety of exercises (e.g., Ferrucci, 1982). Here the exercise "the pie" (Yeomans, 1974) is adapted to our mandala example. Following guidelines discussed earlier, the client constructs a mandala that includes representations of various selves. Thought is given to the amount of territory each self has and how the different selves are positioned relative to each other and other components of the mandala. After meditating on the mandala as a whole, the client begins eavesdropping on the selves, imagining the selves are speaking to and interacting with each other. How do they cooperate or conflict? Which are stronger, in what ways? Do any form alliances against others? The client writes down what he observes and learns, and reflects on how similar dynamics occur in daily living. Finally, the client enters into dialogue with the selves, helping them to appreciate and respect each other, resolve conflicts, and find ways to work together for the needs of the selves and the client.

INTERPERSONAL

Generally, the self is formed, developed, taught, and nourished within a complex set of social relationships (Buss, 1980). Hence, the individual cannot be separated from society, and the self does not exist without relationships (Burkitt, 1991; Holdstock, 1996). This is more obvious with the interdependent self than with the independent self, but is basically true of most selves. The two-way interaction between the individual and society is a basic tenet of social psychology. The self is embedded in a variety of relationships, including social, cultural, political, and economic (Holdstock, 1996).

Hence, it is often important to understand the nature and dynamics of the client's culture, family, friends, and other social groups. It may be important to assess the influence of significant and meaningful others on the client's social behavior and on the helping process (Bankoff & Howard, 1992). Behaviorally, the helper is assessing all relevant operant contingencies. Kaplan (1986) argues that the most inclusive need underlying human behavior is for positive self-evaluation. He suggests a reciprocal relationship between social forces and self-referential behaviors, such as self-evaluation and self-protection. The interpersonal is, of course, important in interpersonal counseling, group therapy, family therapy, and therapeutic communities.

The interpersonal component of helping focuses on the client's relationships with others (Duck, 1998; Johnson, 1993). The field of "human relations" involves the interpersonal skills for working and/or playing with others. Human relations topics include communication, conflict resolution, group dynamics, motivation, models/mentors, and group evolution and development. This is important in a variety of settings, including business (Lamberton & Minor, 1995) and education (Gazda et al., 1999).

There are many behavioral skills the helper can aid the client in developing in order to improve interpersonal relations. This includes training related to communication (Fincham et al., 1993; Gottman et al., 1976; Strayhorn, 1977), assertiveness (Alberti & Emmons, 1995; Lange & Jakubowski, 1976), and parenting (Becker, 1971; Patterson, 1975; Patterson & Forgatch, 1987; Schaefer & Briesmeister, 1989; Sloane, 1988).

Most personal-level therapies, such as psychoanalysis and the humanistic therapies, give primary importance to the relationship between therapist and client. The therapeutic relationship can be a vehicle through which the client can work on general and specific relationship issues. This includes how to establish and improve relationships with others. In psychoanalysis, it is assumed that the therapist is often perceived and responded to as if he or she were similar to or symbolic of some significant other, past or present, often a parent. This "transference" results in conflicts, feelings, and thoughts related to the significant other arising in the therapy situation (generalization).

In the person-centered therapy of Rogers (1951, 1961), the therapist tries to establish a relationship based on genuineness, empathy, and unconditional positive regard. The basic tenet is that when the client experiences all these aspects of the relationship, then the client will engage in the process of personal growth and personality change. This can happen when the client takes more responsibility for problems, experiences emotions in a safe and caring situation, accepts aspects of the self that were unacceptable and/or kept out of consciousness, and experiences a general increase in self-esteem.

A good model for the therapeutic relationship, according to Gestalt therapy theory, is the "I-Thou" relationship described by the influential Jewish philosopher Martin Buber (1923). According to Buber, this relationship is a reciprocal dialogue in which one encounters another human being with all of one's being. One has the courage to be oneself in the relationship. In Buber's translated words (p. 112): "Egos appear by setting themselves apart from other egos. Persons appear by entering into relation to other persons." It is assumed that within this dialogue-encounter, self-revelation will gradually occur. The I-Thou relationship is contrasted with an "I-It" relationship in which the other person is approached as an object, tool, or convenience to be used, manipulated, or exploited. Only some Gestalt therapists try to cultivate an I-Thou relationship. Those who do often try to share of themselves as part of the reciprocal relationship (e.g., Shephard, 1970). Thus, the therapist might acknowledge personal problems and attachments that are similar to those of the client. The therapist surrenders the role of therapist to the interpersonal process.

From a transpersonal point of view, the therapeutic relationship is an opportunity for two beings to meet at a level of being prior to and superordinate to their social roles, personal selves, and personal melodramas. While working with the client on the other three levels of being, the integrative helper also recognizes and cultivates the client's transpersonal level of being, in ways described in later chapters. This creates a spaciousness for conscious exploration in which the client can transcend boundaries in consciousness and disengage from the personal melodrama. A therapy session can be a time when clients step out of their lives, take an intermission in the play, catch their breath, re-center, reflect, plan, play, and then reenter. All of this may be thought of and experienced in a religious/spiritual context or not. As a Jewish mystic, Buber proposed the I-Thou relationship as a way of approaching the world in general, people in specific, and ultimately God. Through I-Thou relationships with other people, one finds God, the eternal, great Thou. Similar to this is the Hindu greeting "Namaste," common in Nepal and India, which means, "I greet the spiritual within you."

From a behavioral point of view, there are many ways a good relationship with the client can facilitate behavior modification (Goldstein & Higginbotham, 1991; Linehan, 1988; Rosenfarb, 1992). A good relationship leads to a more accurate and efficient assessment, and better collaboration on choice of goals and strategies of change. It makes the therapy setting and experiences more positive and, therefore, more enjoyable and effective. It creates a situation where the client can more easily express and release various emotions (respondent extinction). A good relationship makes the therapist a more potent model, a source of stronger reinforcers, and a better motivator. Through reinforcement, encouragement, support, and permission, the therapist motivates the client to try new things and comply with the treatment program.

What constitutes a good therapeutic relationship, from all points of view, is well known and detailed in most counseling and psychotherapy texts (e.g., Cormier & Hackney, 1987; Gelso & Fretz, 1992; Martin, 1983). Characteristics of the optimal therapist include being open, warm, permissive, nonjudgmental, unconditionally accepting, nondefensive, genuine, and honest. A good sense of humor is often helpful. By quieting the mind and opening the heart, the integrative helper learns how to listen, be empathic and compassionate, be in the here and now, and fully enter into relationship with the client. Integrative helpers recognize that there are different personal realities; they respect the autonomy and dignity of the client and are vigilant to their own personal and cultural biases and attachments. The helper recognizes the many needs of the client, such as a need for attention, understanding, respect, support, friendship, and/or someone to confide in. The helper learns when to passively accept the client and when to push or confront the client while still accepting. The helper learns various strategies to deal with clients' resistance, such as pushing the client to do something, educating the client about why it should be done, analyzing the resistance, and sometimes going along with the resistance.

From the client's personal-level point of view, the therapy sessions are a challenge to the sense of self, including optimism about potentials and anxiety and attachments regarding change. And it is often through an act of will that the client will participate and cooperate in the change process and/or enter into a relationship with the helper.

WILL

Totally intertwined with the self is the will. The will is the subjective sense of the self's faculty of decision making and acting. In terms of personal-level experience, there is not only a self, but this self periodically acts through the agency of a will. Consider answers to the earlier questions, "How do I experience myself as the actor?" and "What is your experience of the process of willing?" In Conjunctive Psychology, the self and will are very real at the personal level of being. The approach to the will is phenomenological and pragmatic: phenomenological in that the will is approached in terms of the client's experience of the sense of will, pragmatic in that it is practical and effective for the helper to work with the will.

Although there is an enormous Western literature about the self, there is a relatively small, but important, Western literature about the will (e.g., Assagioli, 1973; Deci, 1980; James, 1890; May, 1969; Rank, 1929). William James suggested that will affects behavior by determining what one attends to and holds in consciousness. Hence, developing the behavior of the mind of concentration would facilitate will. Edward Deci defines "will" as the capacity to choose how to satisfy needs, and defines "self-determination" as the process of utilizing one's will. Deci suggests that the energy for willing comes from the need to be competent and self-determining, a position similar to the theory of "mastery motivation" (MacTurk & Mogan, 1995). Assagioli's psychosynthesis is one of the few therapies that gives primary emphasis to the will and the capacity to choose. Exercises focus on making the will strong, skillful, and ethical. And, within NAMAP, there is a small body of research in which "volition" is a main variable (e.g., Kimble & Perlmuter, 1970; Lazarick et al., 1988).

But what about causality and determinism? When the car does not start, we seldom believe the car has willfully chosen not to cooperate. Rather, we usually assume some natural physical explanation. All of our sciences are based on the assumption that deterministic, causal laws explain the state of things and the processes of change. Psychology as a science, and NAMAP in general, assume deterministic laws of human behavior. This book is filled with such examples. But most individuals believe they have free will, at least in some situations. That is, it seems to the individual that there are times when her behavior is not determined and that what happens is her free choice of will. The assumption of free will is critical to the legal system, morality, and many religions and philosophies.

But how can there be free will in a deterministic world? How can the laws suddenly stop being applicable for a short time? How can one will to violate natural laws? Are there deterministic forces that cause willing? Can one will to will? This is the classic philosophical issue of free will versus determinism (Sappington, 1990; Westcott, 1977). Like all the classic issues, there is no agreed upon solution, and the issue is probably not resolvable by mainstream Western, academic, philosophical approaches. The fact that a person senses being volitional does not necessarily mean this is the best causal explanation, for the self readily claims responsibility for events outside its control. And the previous chapter contains examples of people believing incorrectly that they chose to act for certain reasons, when the actions were due to very different forces that they were not aware of. And where is this self that is doing the willing? No philosophical solutions are offered here. In Conjunctive Psychology, we take a pragmatic stance; often the best approach for a helper is to assume volitional capability and to work with the client's will, including responsibility and effort.

An important part of will work is for clients to take responsibility for desired life changes. This does not refer to taking responsibility for things past that cannot be changed, or getting caught up in blame or regrets. Rather, it is a matter of taking responsibility, here and now, for current concerns and related action programs. The helper is a guide and facilitator of change, but the client is responsible for the changes. Being responsible for oneself is a critical part of humanistic therapies, reality therapy, self-help programs, and most spiritual paths. Confronting one's responsibility and will within the contexts of freedom and meaning is also central to existential psychologists. Even when one is trying to surrender to some higher spiritual being or force, it is critical to take responsibility for one's actions, feelings, and thoughts.

"Right effort" is one of the eight components of the Buddhist eightfold path. It emphasizes the importance of taking action and being persistent in one's mental training and daily living. This effort is done in the context of learning how to do things in ways that are mindful, practical, and harmonious. Research has found that reinforcing a person's effort to do something reduces the aversiveness of the effort and thus increases motivation when in similar situations (Eisenberger, 1992). The more such reinforced experiences a person has, as in childhood, the harder and more persistently he may work and the greater preference he may have for keeping busy and active. Relatedly, attribution research has shown that attributing failure to lack of effort often maximizes subsequent persistence (Försterling, 1985).

MOTIVATION TO CHANGE

An important early factor in a change program is "readiness to hear," the ability of a person to recognize that there is a problem or need to change. For many reasons already discussed, it might take a while before the person reaches this point. It is amazing the amount of suffering people endure before they are finally ready to hear.

After the need is recognized and the client accepts responsibility to do something about it, a change program is developed. Then the next step is for the client to actually do what is necessary for change. This step is often very difficult for the person, whether working alone or with a helper. Many people want to change and know what they need to do; but somehow they never have the time or energy to do it. The complexities and melodramas of their lives keep them unnecessarily tied up. In addition, people procrastinate for various reasons, such as fear of failing at change, dislike of the work involved in changing, concern about rejection or resentment toward changes, fear of the consequences of change such as new responsibilities, and fear that changes will result in an unpleasant situation or a situation with great potential for failure (Rorer, 1983).

Thus, the helper often must assess the client's concerns, beliefs, and attachments related to change, and some of these must be addressed before proceeding with the change program. In addition, it is often useful to do an operant behavior analysis of the reinforcement contingencies related to the current behaviors and the proposed new behaviors. Perhaps the person is being reinforced for her current undesirable behaviors by reinforcers such as attention, concern, or sympathy from others. Perhaps others are sabotaging the person's attempts to change. A husband may sabotage his wife's attempt to lose weight because he doesn't want her to become more attractive to other men. A wife may sabotage her husband's plan to curtail his problem drinking; because if he is successful, she feels she will be forced to confront some of her own problem behaviors.

When it is time to change, the helper helps to elicit and/or develop the client's motivation to change. Picking the right time to change is important, such as a time with little conflicting influences or a day of personal significance. The client might make a list of reasons for changing, a list that is posted, reviewed regularly, and altered over time. At the personal level, the helper encourages the client to take responsibility and put forth the needed effort. But this often needs to be coupled with motivational changes at the behavioral level, including drives and incentives, as discussed earlier.

It may be helpful for clients to learn how to reinforce themselves for carrying out the steps of the change program. This could be formalized into a contract, that might involve other people (Mikulas, 1983a; O'Banion & Whaley, 1981; Watson & Tharp, 1997). Related is the importance of social reinforcement. It is often helpful if friends and family of the client are aware of plans for change, and encourage, support, and reward the gradual steps of the change and the maintenance of the change. A support group might be useful. This could be a group the client or helper establishes, or it might be an existing group, such as Alcoholics Anonymous or Weight Watchers. One has to be careful of the trap of becoming too dependent on the group. Many religious and spiritual traditions value the importance of a community in which members help and support each other. This was very important in the early Christian church and many contemporary Christian religions. In Buddhism, the spiritual community (sangha) is one of the jewels or treasures in which practitioners seek refuge.

A major behavioral-level factor of motivation is the delay of reinforcement, the time between the behavior and the reinforcement (Logue, 1995). Short delays of reinforcement usually have a much stronger effect on behavior than long delays. If a person is in an aversive situation, he may get immediate reinforcement for getting out. But if the problem behavior is pleasant, motivation may be an issue. The immediate reinforcing effects of eating a second piece of pie are stronger than the long-term reinforcing effects of weight loss for not eating the second piece. The problem drinker may receive immediate reinforcement from drinking, such as reduction of anxiety or social reinforcement, whereas the long-term disadvantages of excessive drinking do not have as strong an influence. To deal with issues of delay of reinforcement, the helper may need to help the client imagine future consequences or learn to deal gradually with delay of gratification. Behavior modification procedures, such as contingency contracting and aversive counterconditioning, might be used to change the immediate consequences.

Sometimes a change in motivation is sufficient for behavior change. Perhaps the person had the skills but was just not motivated to act before, or the motivation becomes strong enough to overcome other forces (e.g., "Stop smoking now or be dead in a year"). But motivation changes by themselves are usually not sufficient. Rather, there often needs to be a practical plan of action to produce the desired changes. And usually, the best way to do this is through self-control programs.

SELF-CONTROL

Self-control is a major theme of this book, with some of its advantages discussed in the behavior modification chapter. The act of self-control can be described in terms of four interrelated components: awareness, intervention, sense of self, and sense of will (Mikulas, 1986). First, the person is aware of some less preferred behavior and/or sequence of events leading to a less preferred behavior. Then the person utilizes some intervention strategy to stop or alter the less preferred behavior or sequence to this behavior and/or to increase the probability of a desired alternative. And all of this is associated with a sense of self and will as the agent and action of the awareness and intervention.

The awareness component is cultivated through mindfulness training, discussed in the chapter on behaviors of the mind and throughout this book. Mindfulness training helps the client become more aware of problem behaviors and situations, and related factors, and to notice them earlier and earlier in the chain of events. This increases the client's choices and ease of intervention. Additional ways to increase awareness include keeping behavioral records, receiving feedback from others, viewing videotaped feedback (Hung & Rosenthal, 1978; Meharg & Woltersdorf, 1990), and realistically doing a nonharmful variation of the problem behavior over and over while focusing on the behavior and related behaviors. This latter approach is particularly common in the treatment of "nervous habits," such as biting one's fingernails (Azrin & Nunn, 1977).

Following awareness, the client initiates the intervention strategy. This might be getting out of the situation, taking deep breaths, cueing the body to relax, imagining pleasant scenes, imagining the consequences of the undesired behavior, stopping undesired thoughts and replacing them with desired thoughts, saying affirmations, quieting and focusing the mind, switching to a humorous or compassionate psychological set, reinforcing and punishing specific behaviors, or one of many other types of interventions.

Often the intervention is quite active; the individual does something to change the situation and/or her behavior. Other times, the intervention appears more passive; she alters her mental set to be more accepting of the situation, to fight less against the natural or inevitable flow of events (Shapiro & Astin, 1998). The passive approach is most applicable when the person cannot or should not alter the situation. If it is inevitable that she is not going to get what she wants, then she needs to relax and accept that fact, rather than become frustrated or angry. By being accepting rather than angry, the person can more effectively learn from the situation, regroup, and continue pursuing goals.

Very important at the personal level is for clients to believe they have some control over situations, and that through acts of will and self-control strategies they can produce desired changes. And the best way to produce these beliefs is for them to learn to have more self-control and be aware of this mastery. A number of different literatures converge on these conclusions. From attribution research, we know that people generally get greater and more lasting changes in behavior and attitudes if they attribute the changes to themselves, rather than to external agents or special situations (Harvey & Weary, 1981; Winett, 1970). Thus, it is better when clients feel personally responsible for changes, rather than attributing the changes to such things as drugs or the power of the helper.

Related is the literature on "locus of control" (Lefcourt, 1982; Rotter, 1966). A person with an external locus of control perceives events as largely unrelated to his behavior and outside of his control. A person with an internal locus of control perceives positive and negative events as often being consequences of his own willful behavior and thus under his control. A person who is debilitated by beliefs that aversive events are outside his control is sometimes said to be in a state of "learned helplessness" (Peterson et al., 1993). Some people who are classified as being depressive have an external locus of control and/or are in a state of learned helplessness. Post-traumatic stress disorder is usually due to a very aversive and threatening event that is experienced as uncontrollable and/or unpredictable (Foa et al., 1992). On the other hand, if a person believes he has some control over aversive events, these events may be less aversive and stressful and generate less anticipatory anxiety (Lefcourt, 1976; Miller, 1979; Thompson, 1981). Obviously, the helper helps the client develop an internal locus of control and self-control skills to actually influence self and world.

An extensive, broad, and influential body of research and theory centers on Albert Bandura's concept of "self-efficacy" (Bandura, 1997). "Perceived self-efficacy refers to beliefs in one's capabilities to organize and execute the courses of action required to produce given attainments" (p. 3). Note that this is separate from beliefs about what the outcome will be. Self-efficacy beliefs are correlated with courses of action people choose, how much effort they will put forth in different situations, how long they will persevere in the face of obstacles and failures, whether thoughts are self-hindering or self-aiding, how much stress and depression they experience in taxing situations, and their level of accomplishments.

According to Bandura, there are four sources of information that develop and alter self-efficacy beliefs. First is direct mastery experiences in which the individual perceives her capabilities. Second is vicarious experiences in which others' attainments are a source of comparison and motivation. Third is social evaluations, verbal persuasion, and social influence regarding her capabilities. And fourth is changes in biological states and how they are interpreted, which might be related to strength, vulnerability, or capability. Of these four sources, it is the active mastery experiences that produce the strongest and most generalized efficacy beliefs! How various successes and failures affect efficacy beliefs depends on many factors, such as preconceptions of capabilities, perceived difficulty of task, amount of effort expended, amount of external help received, and the particular circumstances of the situation. Skilled efficacy builders help to structure activities for clients in ways that bring success and avoid repeated failure; and emphasis is put on gradual self-improvement rather than triumph over others.

Thus, the message from attribution theory, locus of control, learned helplessness, and self-efficacy is that it is important for people to believe they can do what is required in various situations and thus have more control over what happens. And usually the best way to develop such beliefs is by actually doing things that increase their capabilities and control, such as cultivating and applying self-control strategies. Shapiro and Astin (1998) suggest that one of the greatest fears is of losing control, and one of the strongest motivations is to have control over one's life.

OTHER LEVELS

An important theme of this chapter is that changes at the behavioral level is often the most effective way to produce changes at the personal level! Changing behavior is usually a powerful approach for increasing self-efficacy, internal locus of control, positive self-concept and positive self-esteem, freedom and choice, and general well-being. These changes, in turn, produce greater and longer lasting behavioral changes.

Personal-level changes can produce behavioral changes in many ways, such as changes in goals and in what is reinforcing and motivating. A discrepancy between the perceived self and the ideal self is usually a source of motivation and dukkha, which leads to behaviors to reduce the discrepancy and/or reduce awareness of the discrepancy.

It is often helpful, experientially and conceptually, to distinguish between the personal level and the behavioral level. Particularly important is to recognize that one's behavior is not one's self. "You are not your behavior" is often good advice. Self-esteem can be based on trying to skillfully change situations and behaviors, not on how "successful" the behaviors are along the way. And as clients gradually disidentify with their behaviors, there is a reduction in their attachments to the behaviors, and thus behavior change is easier.

Relative to terms about the self, a few generalizations can be made. The following terms primarily refer to the personal level: self-concept, self-esteem, self-regard, self-respect, self-importance, self-enhancement, and self-actualization. Moving from the personal level to the transpersonal level involves self-transcendence. At the intersection of the personal and behavioral levels are self-efficacy, self-control, and self-determination. And reinforcers at the behavioral level include self-satisfaction and self-accomplishment.

The level error, the tendency to emphasize just one level of being at the expense of effectiveness and/or appropriateness, is common at all levels. Humanistic therapists and psychoanalysts often focus only on the personal level, or part of it such as the self. This often makes the therapy less effective than approaches that include other levels, such as incorporation of behavior modification. An extreme example of the level error is the belief that establishing a specific type of relationship between client and therapist is the necessary and sufficient condition for personal growth and behavior change. Humanistic psychology was at its peak in the middle of the 20th century and then quickly declined because of two level errors. First was not adequately interfacing with approaches dealing with other levels of being, and thus greatly limiting the applicability and effectiveness of humanistic therapy. Second was the rise of transpersonal psychology, which split the humanistic movement in half. The error here was failing to understand the differences and interrelationships between the personal and transpersonal levels. Some tried to squeeze the transpersonal into the personal. Many struggled with the relationships between self-actualization and self-transcendence. For example, why actualize a self that does not really exist or is going to be transcended and left behind? In Conjunctive Psychology, humanistic contributions are honored, valued, and included in their rightful place.

The self manifests at the biological level in many ways. For example, a person's personality or psychological wounds may manifest in ways often noticed by bodyworkers, such as posture, movement, breathing, gestures, and holding parts of the body in unusual ways (Johnson & Grand, 1998). Therapists and researchers working with multiple selves disorder have reported biological changes when a different self appears. This includes changes in brainwaves, handedness, allergic responses, and need for glasses. In addition, cognitive neuroscientists are gradually identifying brain areas that are related to self as object. For example, encoding of memories related to self seems to involve the left frontal cortex, while retrieval of these memories involves the right frontal cortex (Craik et al., 1999).

Beliefs in controllability (e.g., locus of control, self-efficacy) influence biological health (Shapiro & Astin, 1998). When a person encounters potential stressors in life, the less the person feels control over the situation, the greater the stress and the greater the impairment of the immune system (Bandura, 1997; Lefcourt, 1976; Miller, 1979; Thompson, 1981). There are lots of opportunities for a self-fulfilling prophecy here. For example, a person has some poor health, which leads to a self-concept of poor health, which leads to a belief of little control over health, which results in more stress and fewer efforts at doing things to improve health, which leads to poorer health, and so on.

Periodically, there have been research reports of biological correlates of volition that precede the subjective experience of willing (e.g., Libet et al., 1983). This raises the following question: What is the nature of will if a technician, using neurophysiological information, could identify what choice a person will make before the person consciously makes the choice? One possibility, according to Libet and associates, is that the person could consciously veto voluntary acts that were unconsciously initiated. Self-control here is the choice not to act. And what if this choice was also predictable?

Interpersonal relationships also impact on biological health. For example, family and friends may model, reinforce, and encourage healthy or unhealthy behaviors. Research has revealed that social support is related to beneficial effects on the cardiovascular, endocrine, and immune system (Uchino et al., 1996). Ways this might happen include providing emotional support and helping to deal with potential stress. Overall "people supported by close relationships with friends, family, or fellow members of church, work, or other support groups are less vulnerable to ill health and premature death" (Myers, 2000, p. 62). For example, religious involvement is associated with living longer (McCullough et al., 2000).

The interpersonal is also a major vehicle to the transpersonal, as was suggested for the I-Thou relationship. By gradually and experientially understanding his embeddedness in social/cultural entities, a person can gradually disidentify with a sense of a separate and perhaps alienated personal self. Of all the world's religions, Judaism is one that gives particular importance to the family and society. For example, the Jewish commandments include not killing, stealing, and lying, which are found in many religions; but they also include honoring one's father and mother and maintaining social harmony with the group. Karma yoga is a spiritual path in which one tries to live and act from an orientation of sacrifice and selfless service. One tries to act with precision and awareness and without attachments, as one serves and helps others.

Finally, as the discussion shifts to the transpersonal level, an important point needs to be stressed: There is no problem with the existence of a personal-level self. It is a major mistake of many people to think that the self must be undone or killed before the transpersonal can emerge. The personal level self should always be valued and worked with in ways discussed above. Transpersonal issues relate to attachments to this self and beliefs that one's personal reality is all there is.

SUMMARY

The self is the center of the personal reality: the observer of perceptions and memories, the thinker of thoughts, and the agent of willful decision making and acting. The self as object includes the thoughts, memories, attitudes, and feelings one has toward one's self, the domains of self-concept and self-esteem.

It is sometimes useful to think of a person as having more than one self and that these other selves come into existence in different situations. Often this is no problem, and it may actually be helpful to the person. Sometimes the selves are in conflict, and this conflict must be reduced and/or the selves integrated into a more holistic healthier self. The extreme problematic situation is multiple selves disorder.

The self develops in a complex set of cultural and social relationships, the interpersonal domain. There are dramatic cultural and gender differences among selves, such as the independent self versus the interdependent self, which relate to how the self is enmeshed in the interpersonal. Once a self is formed, there is often resistance to change, based on self-attachments.

Therapies for the self involve working with various combinations of self as object, integration of self, restructuring the self, self-related attachments, and transcendence of the self. This is the primary domain of humanistic therapies and psychoanalysis. Comparing the self with an ideal self may provide motivation and direction; it may also elicit anxiety or depression. When problematical, it may be necessary to change the ideal self and/or how the person responds to the discrepancy, the latter being a primary focus of Buddhist therapy.

The will is the subjective sense of the self's decision making and acting. Therapies emphasize taking responsibility for one's life and exerting sufficient effort to do what needs to be done. Sometimes the best strategy is to actively do something; sometimes it is best to be more passive and accepting.

Factors related to the motivation to change include readiness to hear, reasons for change, barriers to change, and reinforcement for changing and not changing. Delay of reinforcement is sometimes important here and in developing self-control.

There are two very important dynamics of psychology that helpers need to remember, put into practice, and confirm for themselves. The first is that changes at the biological and/or behavioral levels is often the most effective way to produce changes at the personal level, such as in self-concept and self-esteem. The second is that one of the most important factors in biological and psychological health is the person's belief in personal control, that one can do what is required in various situations. And the best way to develop this belief is by doing things that actually give the person such control, such as developing self-control skills and strategies. Put together, these principles emphasize getting out and doing something.

Author's Reflections

In the United States, college students of the 1990s were much more passive than students of previous decades. They asked fewer questions and were less interested in affecting their own education. They were less involved in social issues, political concerns, and personal/spiritual growth. They were less engaged in the world. This detachment may have serious long-range effects on their health and happiness. What should be happening in education to deal with such issues? How will the next group of students be different?

Currently, boredom is an epidemic in the United States. This is often hard for some people in other parts of the world to understand, since we have so much stuff and types of entertainment and distraction. But when college students in the United States are polled about their concerns and problems, money is on the top of the list and boredom is number two. A major cause of boredom is passivity. If people sit back and rely on the world to entertain them, they are vulnerable to boredom and blame the world for it. It is important for such people to take more responsibility for their psychological states and to be more actively involved in the world. Rather than relying on the world for entertainment and answers, they should take what the world offers and think about it, work with it, and play with it.

Most people are readily lost in the contents of their minds, including self as object. Hence, it is difficult for a self to be an observer of what it believes to be the self, when the person is pulled into the self-related contents. This is resolvable through meditation or some equivalent practice. Through meditation one gradually disengages from the contents of the mind and stands back and objectively observes the contents, including what one took to be the self. From this position, it is easier to change the self and discover self-related attachments.

THOUGHT QUESTIONS

The questions and self-meditations at the beginning of the chapter are powerful thought questions and devices to lead to experiential knowing of the self. As mentioned earlier, thought questions in this book with numbers in parentheses are questions from students in a Conjunctive Psychology course.

(1.) How can you envision the "questions and self-meditations" section being relevant for therapists? How could we incorporate this into therapy?

2. The Buddhist philosopher Nagarjuna asks (Batchelor, 2000): Am I already here before I see and taste and feel? If not, how could I see and taste and feel? How can I know if I am already here or not? Can the seer taste? Can the taster feel?

3. Consider two hypothetical clients with the same diagnosis (of your choice). Describe how their therapies would differ if one client were primarily independent, and the other primarily interdependent.

(4.) Does not each person have both independent and interdependent characteristics? Does the helper look at where the problem is, or is it a classification of the person and not the problem?

5. Carl Rogers claimed that the major factor affecting self-esteem is being accepted and respected by significant others. What does this suggest about the interrelationships between the personal and behavioral levels?

6. Describe a case in which self-esteem is best altered by personal-level therapies, as opposed to behavioral and biological interventions. Why is it so in this case?

7. How would you assess a client's ideal self or selves?

8. What are two of your ideal selves? What are the advantages and disadvantages of them?

(9.) What are the behavioral implications for someone who views himself as a "trouble maker?" What mistakes might that person continually make, just because that is how he defines himself?

10. How would you assess a client's self-related attachments?

11. How would you assess a client's different selves or subpersonalities?

12. List two or three of your subpersonalities. Give them names or titles.

13. Give an example, different from the one in the chapter, where it is desirable to have different selves.

14. What is a possible cause of multiple selves disorder, other than abuse as a child?

15. Give a detailed example of personal psychosynthesis for a hypothetical case.

(16.) In what kinds of situations would you work on transcending the self, as opposed to continuing self-related work? Where do you draw that line?

17. If you are not the contents of your mind, who are you?

18. How would developing the I-Thou relationship be part of marriage counseling?

(19.) When a client's locus of control is almost exclusively external, how might the integrative helper increase self-efficacy?

20. Describe the components of your own new "will therapy."

21. How could belonging to a support group help and hinder a person's behavior change and biological health?

22. How does a person's sense of self and will affect biological health?

TRANSPERSONAL LEVEL

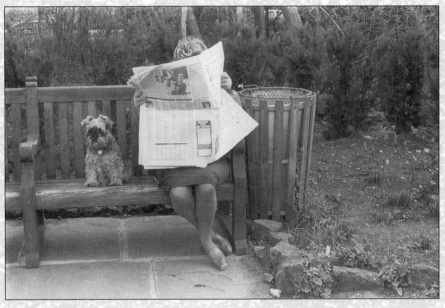

Photo by Benita Mikulas

THE TRANSPERSONAL
DOMAIN

The transpersonal level includes forces and domains of being that are superordinate to and/or prior to the self-centered personal reality. Whereas the personal level focuses on specific contents of consciousness, the transpersonal is more concerned with the processes of consciousness, and eventually consciousness per se as an aspect of the fundamental ground. The personal level emphasizes working with a specific self (or selves), while the transpersonal is more concerned with the dynamic forces that produce a sense of self, the field in which various selves may arise, and domains of being which are not self-centered.

In Conjunctive Psychology, "transpersonal" refers to how the individual is embedded in forces and processes that create and support the individual. Consider the biological level. According to contemporary astronomy, all the material used to build a human body was originally part of a star. Hence, the material could be traced from star to body by principles of physics, chemistry, and biology. DNA could be traced across generations and many people as it leads to the blueprint for constructing a particular body from this material. Most of the body is continually breaking down and being replaced, part by part. To do this, the body consumes various plants and/or animals to provide construction pieces. The lives of these various plants and animals could be traced before they are consumed. And energy for the body comes from the sun. So this energy could be traced from the sun to the body through many intermediaries. Earlier, it was discussed how the body is composed of fields of EMR (electromagnetic radiation) embedded in other fields of EMR. The point is that the body is not a fixed separate entity. Rather, it is a continually changing complex of processes embedded in a field of other processes.

Similarly, at the behavioral level the body's behaviors are not occurring in a vacuum. Rather, many behaviors are a result of the forces described by psychology, sociology, and anthropology. Specific behaviors could be traced across time and cultures, such as particular thoughts, verbal expressions, and fashions. And at the personal level, it was earlier discussed how the individual self is totally embedded in the interpersonal.

Everywhere we look, we see the interconnectedness of things. The field of ecology is based on this premise. For example, people wanted more hamburgers, which led to clearing of rain forests in order to have land to raise more cows; and the destruction of trees has affected the weather of the whole earth.

Hence, the transpersonal is concerned with how the individual is embedded in that which is greater than the individual ("trans" = "beyond"). Some readers may understand this as how the individual is embedded in nature and natural laws. Others may include cosmic principles, such as karma or the relationship between the individual and God. In this book is discussed transpersonal psychology, but there are many other transpersonal disciplines, such as transpersonal anthropology, transpersonal education, transpersonal social work, transpersonal medicine, transpersonal art, and transpersonal business (Boucouvalas, 1999).

In Conjunctive Psychology, transpersonal psychology is the study of the nature of the transpersonal level of being and how this level relates to psychological aspects of other levels of being. This includes theories, practices, and research. All major Eastern psychologies give prime emphasis to cultivation of, awareness of, and uncovering of the transpersonal level.

In the West, transpersonal psychology was slow to develop. Some of the first Western psychologists to address the transpersonal and use a term like "transpersonal" include William James, Carl Jung, and Roberto Assagioli. But it was not until the second half of the 20th century that transpersonal psychology came together as a branch of Western psychology (Boorstein, 1996; Rowan, 1993; Scotton et al., 1996; Tart, 1990; Walsh & Vaughan, 1993). The field includes ways to measure and research transpersonal constructs (Braud & Anderson, 1998; MacDonald et al., 1995; 1999a, 1999b) and implications for therapy (Cortright, 1997; Nelson, 1994; Vaughan, 1995). Based on a survey of many definitions of transpersonal psychology, Lajoie and Shapiro (1992, p. 91) suggest that "Transpersonal psychology is concerned with the study of humanity's highest potential, and with the recognition, understanding, and realization of unitive, spiritual, and transcendent states of consciousness."

Currently, NAMAP basically does not include transpersonal psychology in its programs, texts, or other literature. In the American Psychological Association, transpersonal psychology is officially a subset of humanistic psychology (the level error).

The goal of most Western psychotherapists is to help the client cope better with his or her life. A helper cannot eliminate all the suffering from a client's life, but he or she can help the person be better able to cope with or accept the suffering. Eastern psychologies and transpersonal psychology suggest we can do better than that. They argue that beyond coping and accepting there is the possibility of a fundamental liberation from suffering. Whether and how such liberation occurs is an extraordinary challenge to Western therapies. Ram Dass (Richard Alpert) suggests that "Western psychotherapy rearranges the furniture in the room. Eastern techniques help you get out of the room." Transpersonal therapy helps the client discover freedom, equanimity, peace of mind, and love.

KNOWING

It is heuristic to differentiate three different types of knowing: sensory, conceptual, and insight. Sensory knowing is the experiential knowing based on the senses. If you want to know what a banana tastes like, it is usually best to eat a banana;

conceptual descriptions from others are not sufficient. Conceptual knowing is based on concepts, words, and ideas, the knowing of philosophy and logic. Universities in the United States are primarily devoted to conceptual knowledge. Insight knowing refers to nonsensory, nonconceptual understanding that arises in consciousness. It is converted into conceptual knowledge when it is thought about or described. Insight includes some forms of intuition; Buddhist "prajna," which is immediately experienced intuitive wisdom; and the counsel of the Christian Holy Spirit. Psychotherapy sometimes works by generating this type of insight (Bohart & Wugalter, 1991).

Vipassana meditation is called insight meditation because the cultivation of mindfulness via vipassana leads to insight knowing. For example, you can conceptually know that everything changes, and this knowledge may not affect your being. But when you mindfully experience the impermanence of things in an insightful way, then your being is usually significantly altered. You are less likely to become attached to things as a source of happiness.

Ken Wilber (1996b) provides the best discussion of these three different types of knowing, described in terms of the eye of flesh, the eye of mind, and the eye of contemplation (following St. Bonaventure and Hugh of St. Victor). According to Wilber, a comprehensive understanding of reality must involve the knowledge from all three eyes. Many problems in psychology, science, philosophy, and religion result from applying the wrong eye and/or reducing all "acceptable" knowledge to what is revealed by a single eye. Wilber argues that each eye has its own set of injunctions: if you want to know this, you must do this (e.g., eat the banana, follow this mathematical proof, practice meditation). The truthfulness of what one comes to know is verified by others who have followed the same injunctions. This is similar to the earlier argument about state-specific sciences.

At the biological and behavioral levels, the eyes of flesh and mind are quite adequate. But at the personal and transpersonal levels, we also need the eye of contemplation (Hart et al., 2000). To fully understand one's self requires contemplation of the self, guided by injunctions, such as the questions at the beginning of the last chapter. And the transpersonal level is only truly understood through the eye of contemplation. To accomplish this, one follows a set of injunctions that lead to insight about the transpersonal (e.g., Flickstein, 2001; Mikulas, 1987; Savitripriya, 1991; Walsh, 1999). These insights are substantiated by others who have followed similar injunctions. The Zen master can verify the insights of one who practices Zen meditation (zazen).

Translation between different types of knowing is often problematical. When insights about the transpersonal are translated into conceptual forms, they may not make sense or may appear paradoxical. Understanding the transpersonal is impaired by demanding data that come only through the eyes of flesh and mind. Earlier we discussed two unresolved philosophical issues: the mind-body problem and free will versus determinism. Wilber suggests that both are resolvable only via the eye of contemplation. But the resolution does not translate into conceptual knowledge in a way that resolves the philosophical conceptual issues.

So what do we learn about the transpersonal level through the eye of contemplation? First, reality is apprehended directly and immediately, not via words and concepts. This apprehension is outside time and space and not distorted in the ways previously described for perceptions and thoughts. Second, what is apprehended is a sense of unity, total interconnectedness. This knowing is not the dualistic knowing of the personal level. Subject and object disappear into the nondual unity.

This discussion is, of course, conceptual and not the best way to know about the transpersonal. And it is not necessary for the integrative helper to believe any of it. More important for the helper is the client's development related to the transpersonal.

DEVELOPMENT

In Western transpersonal psychology, individual development is often described as potentially going through three basic stages: prepersonal, personal, and transpersonal. Prepersonal occurs early in life, before one has developed a pervasive sense of self and before one becomes lost in the personal reality.

The personal stage of development begins as one acquires a sense of a personal self and the issues of the personal level of being begin to become prominent. Teenagers in the United States are generally in the middle of the personal stage, often very self-centered and driven by self-concerns of identity, independence, and popularity. Some people will never develop beyond the personal stage.

But many people are motivated to continue their development into the transpersonal stage. For example, a common cause of motivation occurs when a person discovers that what he thought would bring fulfillment and happiness in life is just not working. In commercial America, many people seek happiness or status by collecting more and more stuff (e.g., clothes, cars, electronic gadgets, money) and by living a lifestyle dictated by advertisers and the media. When these do not provide the fulfillment expected and promised, the person may have a personal crisis (e.g., midlife crisis, existential crisis) and/or seek what more there is to life, including the transpersonal.

Some people are motivated toward the transpersonal by existential and spiritual yearnings, anxiety, feelings of isolation, a search for meaning, or a desire for a deeper connection and greater coherence between self and world. Others have had experiences (e.g., peak, flow, mystical, psychic) that they perceive as a taste of the transpersonal that they wish to explore further.

Is there a basic, perhaps universal, form of motivation that pushes or pulls evolution and/or individual development toward the transpersonal? Some transpersonal theorists, humanists, existentialists, and religious philosophers would say there is (e.g., de Chardin, 1959; Wilber, 1995). Bill Wilson, the founder of Alcoholics Anonymous, believed that the alcoholic's reliance on alcohol was a distorted search for some kind of transpersonal experience. Carl Jung felt this way about some of his clients and told Wilson that the only cure for alcoholism is a transpersonal cure. One reason for the current popularity of 12-step programs, such as Alcoholics Anonymous, is the inclusion of the transpersonal component.

After a person has adequately resolved many of the issues at the personal level, then he can progress to the transpersonal. It can be harmful and inefficient to try prematurely to transcend the personal level and/or engage in some transpersonal practices. A person coming out of an ego-shattering divorce may need to work on his self-concept and self-esteem, not have his very essence of self challenged. A person with a very fragile sense of self and many repressed aspects of self can be overwhelmed by meditation practices that open the gates of consciousness, letting repressed material in at a rate such that it cannot be profitably assimilated.

Development from the personal stage to the transpersonal stage involves disidentifying with the self of the personal level as the totality of one's being. It involves getting free from being lost in the melodrama of the personal reality, where one's happiness depends on the plot of the melodrama and what the script says one needs to be happy. This does not mean that the personal-level self and related constructs disappear or lose their functional usefulness. They are simply added to as one uncovers the transpersonal level of being.

Much of existentialism is concerned with the border of the personal and transpersonal levels of being, and during development, an individual may enter existential domains on the way to the transpersonal. At the existential level, she comes to see the limitations, arbitrariness, and meaninglessness of much of culturally conditioned personal realities. She then often tries to find or establish some meaning and authenticity in her life. At the existential level, one encounters a fundamental source of suffering (dukkha) based on a feeling of isolation, not being related to the whole. All of this may be thought of in terms of a self (e.g., Kierkegaard) or not (e.g., Sartre), and from a perspective that is theistic (e.g., Kierkegaard) or atheistic (e.g., Nietzsche). Existential psychotherapy focuses on some of the issues encountered at the existential level, such as freedom, isolation, meaninglessness, and death (Yalom, 1980). This approach often includes cultivating a here-and-now awareness of one's being and experience, which fits the mindfulness theme of Buddhism and Conjunctive Psychology. A possible trap is to be caught in existential domains and not continuing development, a trap responsible for considerable anxiety and many suicides. Fortunately, the concerns of the existential stage are resolved at the transpersonal stage. And one can find transpersonal components in the philosophies and experiences of existentialists, such as Heidegger. The integrative helper ensures that the client has a guide for traveling through existential domains and into the transpersonal.

How to uncover the transpersonal is discussed in the next chapter. Here are some of the results of such development. First, one moves into a broader conscious domain and uncovers a very sane, awake, clear, and centered aspect of being that is particularly open to insight knowing. During the gradual transition from personal to transpersonal, one periodically has an experiential sense of this calm and clear domain, which gradually provides a frame of reference relative to how much one is lost in the melodrama of the personal reality. Second, the mind becomes free from unnecessary service to the personal-level self. Klein (1988) distinguishes between psychological memory of the personal stage and functional memory of the transpersonal stage. Psychological memory recalls constantly, as a means to perpetuate the sense of self, while functional memory appears spontaneously as needed. Relatedly, when thinking is freed from memory, it is more creative. "Creative thinking never begins with the already known, a representation. It is born and dies in openness and merely uses functional memory for its expression" (Klein, 1988, p. 50).

Third, one is experientially more in the here and now. At the personal stage of development, one is seldom in the here and now; much of the time one is lost in memories of the past or anticipations of the future. But at the transpersonal stage, there is much less of this remembering and fantasizing; and when it does appropriately occur, one does not get pulled into and lost in it. Rather, one has the experience of being in the here and now with a mind that is planning or remembering. This is the distinction between being lost in the contents of the mind and being an observer of the contents.

The fourth result of transpersonal development is that one finds peace of mind and fulfillment that are independent of the events in the personal-level melodrama. And the fifth result is that one's behavior becomes motivated primarily by appropriateness and compassion. This behavior is more spontaneous, obvious, harmonious, and selfless.

Finally, there is an important trap relative to the development discussed above, a trap Wilber (1996b) calls the "pre/trans fallacy." This is where the prepersonal is confused with the transpersonal, since they are both not personal. Or in the developmental sequence prerational, rational, and transrational, the prerational is confused with the transrational, since both are nonrational. Wilber provides many examples of the pre/trans fallacy. In one form of the fallacy, transpersonal states are reduced to prepersonal states and thus explained away. This was the position of Freud and is a common belief in NAMAP. For Freud, development ends in the personal stage and apparent transpersonal development is regression back to earlier prepersonal stages—hence, Freud's negative attitude toward religion and spirituality. In the second form of the fallacy, prepersonal states are elevated to transpersonal status. People committing this fallacy include Jung and some transpersonal theorists. Currently, many people are eliciting prepersonal-based experiences that they think are transpersonal in nature. For example, a prepersonal memory might be pulled from the unconscious and then thought to be a transpersonal vision.

Now consider how this development toward the transpersonal seems to the personal-level self.

PERSONAL VIEW

There are many ways people have thought about and described uncovering the transpersonal level of being. Metzner (1998) discusses 10 such metaphors: awakening from the dream of "reality," uncovering the veils of illusion, moving from captivity to liberation, being purified by inner fire, emerging from darkness to light, progressing from fragmentation to wholeness, journeying to the place of vision and power, returning to the source, dying and being reborn, and unfolding the tree of our life.

Of these, the metaphor of awakening from the dream of "reality" is one of the most common. The word "buddha" means "awakened one", and the historical

Buddha did not claim to be other than a human being, just one of many who awoke. When we are asleep and dreaming, the dream can seem very real; it is the reality we live in. Then when we awake, we move into another domain of consciousness and realize the dream was a product of the mind. Similarly, as we move into the personal stage of development, we gradually fall asleep into the dream of the personal reality. When we later awaken from this dream, we realize the personal reality was a product of the mind. There is no problem with the personal reality, and it maintains its functions. But we realize there is more, and we are less vulnerable to what happens in the dream of the personal reality. For most people, the process of awakening from the personal reality is a gradual process. We wake a little, then fall back asleep, then wake again, and so on. Gradually we stay awake longer and do not fall as deeply asleep.

The way an individual experiences, conceptualizes, and expresses the transpersonal, through the other levels of being, is a function of the individual's culture, personality, and vocation, among other factors. Across cultures and time, we find the transpersonal described and expressed in many forms, including art, science, and philosophy. Beautiful and powerful descriptions are found in paintings, dance, poetry, folk tales, mathematics, physics, philosophy, psychology, and religion.

For most people, the transpersonal has a religious or spiritual flavor to it, and all the world's major religions are intersections of the transpersonal with cultural beliefs and practices. Hence, some readers may prefer to substitute "spiritual" for "transpersonal," and "spiritual work" for "transpersonal development." Most clients consider spirituality or religion to be important or very important in their lives (cf. Bergin, 1991). Thus, the integrative helper must recognize and respect the client's religious views and understand how to approach the transpersonal from this orientation. As Bergin (1991, p. 401) concludes, "there is a spiritual dimension of human experience with which the field of psychology must come to terms more assiduously. If psychologists could understand it better than they do now, they might contribute toward improving both mental and social conditions."

This association with religion has made the transpersonal very problematical for NAMAP, since religion is still generally a taboo topic. However, the transpersonal need not be conceptualized or approached from a religious orientation. In fact, the transpersonal is prior to any particular set of beliefs or experiences.

Related to awakening is a very important fact: the personal self cannot awaken, cannot move into the transpersonal, cannot become enlightened, etc! The reason is that awakening involves disidentifying with this self and moving beyond ("trans") the personal. The self merges into the unity of the transpersonal. This is a problem for the self, which fights for its existence and perhaps would like to add "awakened one" to its personal credentials. So the self converts the awakening into a self adventure. Now it is the self that is awakening and transcending itself, which, of course, is impossible. This is a very common trap. To do this, the self deceives itself that it is developing transpersonally or spiritually when it is really strengthening egocentricity through transpersonal practices (Hendlin, 1983; Tungpa, 1973). There are many opportunities for delusion here, such as confusing the prepersonal with the transpersonal and exaggerating one's spiritual accomplishments. This is why a guide who can recognize these delusions and traps is often helpful—some would say necessary.

The second very important fact is that the transpersonal level of being is already always present! It is not something to be constructed in the future; it is present now. We must simply awaken to its existence. Said another way, the highest transpersonal/spiritual levels cannot be obtained. If they could, they would be limited in time, occurring after some time, and separable from oneself since they would be something one obtains. Instead, these higher levels are one without a second, unlimited, and outside of time and space. Therefore, they are always already here. We are already awakened, even if the self does not realize it. This is the type of paradox that arises when conceptualizing the transpersonal rather than seeing it through the eye of contemplation. In the words of Ramana Maharshi, "There is no greater mystery than this—that being the reality we seek to gain reality" (Godman, 1985, p. 55).

The above discussion has emphasized the awakening metaphor. An alternative way of conceptualizing much of this chapter is in terms of levels of consciousness, building on the earlier discussion of states of consciousness.

LEVELS OF CONSCIOUSNESS

Domain of consciousness A is said to be a higher level than domain of consciousness B, if A includes all of B and more—that is, if B is a subset of A. Here we consider four levels of consciousness that cover the transpersonal domain. There are many, far more detailed maps of higher levels of consciousness (Alexander & Langer, 1990; Buddhaghosa, 1975; Washburn, 1995; Wilber, 1995).

The first level is consensus waking consciousness, the normal awake consciousness of the personal level of being. This consciousness is often dualistic in that there is a self perceiving an object. The two depend on each other and bring each other into existence.

The second level of consciousness is the witness level. This level arises as we disengage from the contents of the mind. In the first level, we are readily pulled into the contents of the mind and quickly lost. Then, through practices such as mindfulness meditation, we step back from the contents and become a witness of them without getting lost in them. We become an objective observer of our body, behavior, and mind. The witness level is readily accessible to many people and facilitates behavior change and personal growth, for reasons discussed earlier relative to mindfulness. While cultivating the witness, we often move back and forth between the first two levels of consciousness. Note that the witness level is still dualistic; there is a witness observing things, but the witness is quite different from the self and is an observer of the self.

The third level of consciousness is the unity/void level. On the unity side, the distinction between me and not me disappears and the individual has insight knowing of the unity of all things. This is usually accompanied by experiences of peace, bliss, and understanding. There is also usually a change in values and ethics. If everything is part of the unity, how could a person intentionally hurt another person or do something to profit herself at the expense of another? Moral behavior is more obvious and less effortful.

The other side of unity is the void or nothingness (no thingness). There is no unity without the void; they are like two sides of the same coin. Entrance into the void can be very frightening and/or liberating. A guide here is often very important.

Although the self and witness dissolve into the unity/void, this level is still subtly dualistic; there is still some experience of the unity or the void. When this last duality is transcended, we enter the fourth level of consciousness, consciousness without an object (Merrell-Wolff, 1973). This is pure nondualistic consciousness, an aspect of the fundamental ground of the transpersonal. Nothing that can be said about this level is true, for all language and conceptual knowledge is dualistic. For example, we cannot say this level is formless, for that implies a distinction between form and formless, which are both included and transcended. And it implies some observer of form or formlessness. We cannot say this level is inside or outside of time and space, because that is based on the duality of inside/outside. We can only know this level through the eye of contemplation.

Experience and direct knowledge of the third and perhaps the fourth level of consciousness are what is meant by "enlightenment" (White, 1995) and "mysticism" (Ellwood, 1999; Stace, 1960), in the strict sense of these terms. The first taste of enlightenment is usually very brief. Further enlightenments last longer and have greater impact on the other levels of being. For Buddhists, yogis, Sufis, and mystics of all traditions, enlightenment is the goal and purpose of personal existence.

In Wilber's developmental model (1995), he suggests four stages of transpersonal development: psychic, subtle, causal, and nondual. These correspond to four types of mysticism: nature mysticism (mystical union with the realm of nature), deity mysticism (centering on the form of divinity), formless mysticism (the unmanifest causal realm), and nondual mysticism (the fourth level of consciousness described above.)

The integrative helper does not have to understand or believe in higher levels of consciousness, but he or she must respect the importance of these to many people and be aware that there are related literatures and practices that might be useful to some clients. Also, many people who try to achieve enlightenment fall into the trap, discussed above, of the self doing things for the self to become enlightened; this cannot happen. The better way is to follow basic practices that improve one's life at all levels of being and open the way for enlightenment to emerge naturally. This is the topic of the next chapter.

SUMMARY

The transpersonal level is concerned with the forces and processes that create and support the individual and the personal reality, how the individual is embedded in that which is greater than the individual. It includes processes of consciousness and consciousness itself. It is often conceptualized from a spiritual perspective, but this is not necessary.

There are three distinctly different ways of knowing: sensory, conceptual, and insight. A comprehensive psychology or cosmology must include what is learned from all three. The transpersonal level is best understood by insight knowing, which may lead to significant transformation in a person's whole being.

Development goes from prepersonal to personal, and then perhaps to transpersonal. In the personal stage of development, the individual's personal reality is the totality of reality. Uncovering the transpersonal level of being involves disidentifying with the personal reality, a process that often feels something like waking up from a dream. The personal reality, including the personal-level self, remains in existence with important functions. But one discovers there is much more! The personal-level self cannot wake up, since awakening involves transcending the self. The trap of the self trying to awaken itself has currently caught thousands of people.

Uncovering the transpersonal level of being leads to clarity and sanity, being more in the here and now, motivation based on appropriateness and compassion, and behavior that is more spontaneous and harmonious. It also results in understanding, peace of mind, and fulfillment, which many people, perhaps everyone, seek in one form or another.

There are many detailed maps of different levels of consciousness. The four levels discussed in the chapter are consensus waking consciousness, witness level, unity/void, and consciousness without an object. The latter two are transpersonal levels that include enlightenment. The witness level is the transition level, a door to the transpersonal.

AUTHOR'S REFLECTIONS

The transpersonal level of being is a significant part of most of the world's psychologies (e.g., Eastern, African, Native American), but transpersonal psychology has not fared well in NAMAP. A major reason is its association with religion and new age silliness. In addition, as a movement in the United States, it has been too provincial and filled with examples of the pre/trans fallacy.

Most important, relative to the themes of the book, is that the transpersonalists have not done a good job interfacing the transpersonal with other levels of being. (There are numerous important exceptions to this, many of which are referenced in this and the next chapter.) For this reason, Ken Wilber no longer considers himself a transpersonal philosopher. He is now an "integral" theorist. Relatedly, a goal of this book, and Conjunctive Psychology in general, is to make the transpersonal more "reasonable" and accessible, and to explore interactions with other levels of being. Much work needs to be done here.

When talking about different levels of consciousness, I usually begin with consensus waking consciousness, stressing the types of points covered in the earlier chapter on conscious personal reality. I spend most of the time on the witness level, since this is the next step for most people, and a level most can understand. Movement into the witness level can be accomplished by many people, probably most people reading this book. The last two levels, unity/void and consciousness without an object, I touch on only briefly because they are harder to understand and become a little too mystical and esoteric for many. But there always are numbers of people who have had brief experiences related to these two levels.

This book is primarily conceptual knowledge, but I have included a number of activities that can lead to other types of knowing, as listed at the end of the preface. The questions and self-meditations that begin the last chapter form a very powerful example.

THOUGHT QUESTIONS

1. What is your understanding and description of the transpersonal level of being?
(2.) Given that the transpersonal can only be awkwardly and often paradoxically put into conceptual forms, should it be regarded as fundamentally incommensurable with the NAMAP approach?
3. What are some of the practical implications of the level error of making transpersonal psychology a subset of humanistic psychology?
(4.) How, in addition to meditation, can one access the eye of contemplation?
5. Describe a personal example of insight knowing.
(6.) What is the implication of different modes of knowing having different modes of proof?
(7.) Why are different types of knowing important when dealing with a client?
8. When would it be appropriate to focus therapy primarily at the existential level?
9. Based on your knowledge of the personal level, elaborate on Klein's distinction between psychological memory and functional memory.
10. Discuss two of the 10 metaphors for uncovering the transpersonal level, other than the awakening metaphor.
11. Describe enlightenment within a religion of your choice.
12. How can the transpersonal level be already present, yet unknown?
13. What would motivate you to uncover the transpersonal?
(14.) When a client has fallen into the trap of self-deceit, incorrectly believing he or she has developed transpersonally, how might the integrative helper approach the task of dissolving this delusion?
15. What are the practical implications of the pre-trans fallacy for the integrative helper?

THE WAY BEYOND

CHAPTER

11

Self-centeredness is a key distinction between the personal and transpersonal levels, and attachments to the self are major obstacles to transpersonal development. Therefore, consider this self from a transpersonal point of view.

First, the self is not always around. For example, during dreamless sleep there is no self, hence, we cannot base a continuous existence on this self. In sports, an athlete may lose the self during periods of peak performance, such as being "in the zone" (Murphy & White, 1978, 1995). The self may disappear when we become absorbed in something, such as a sensory experience or intense concentration meditation. Thus, there may be no self when we are absorbed in music or in a contemplative/concentration meditation on Jesus. More subtle is the absence of a self in some situations when a desire has just been fulfilled, a project completed, or in the space between thoughts. Sexual intercourse as a spiritual practice involves two beings merging into one.

Transpersonal practices often involve mindfully exploring this self. For example, when one is upset, this is a cue to look for exactly who is upset. One eventually finds that there is no constant, separate entity that is a self. Rather, there is a flowing set of phenomena and processes, including perceptions, thoughts, and attachments. Buckminster Fuller stated, "I seem to be a verb."

Two ways to get beyond the self are the external path and the internal path, which may lead to extrovertive mysticism or introvertive mysticism, respectively (Stace, 1960). In the external path, one surrenders one's self to one's family, group, or God. In love and service to others, one transcends self-centeredness. In the internal path, one turns in on one's consciousness and moves through the self to the transpersonal. For example, in psychodynamic depth approaches, one goes deep inside, past the personal and the repressed, until a fundamental sense of presence or essence emerges (Almaas, 1986; Cortright, 1997; Davis, 1999). The external path and internal path both lead to transpersonal domains. Different paths are, of course, appropriate for different people at different times.

The existence of the subjective self depends on the subject-object duality. The self thus vanishes when one of these dissolves into the other. Thus, as mentioned above, the self disappears when one becomes absorbed in perceptions and/or actions. This is related to what Csikszentmihalyi (1990) refers to as "flow," which he considers to be the optimal experience and criterion of happiness. Common characteristics of flow include a chance one can complete a worthwhile and/or difficult task, clear goals and immediate feedback, a sense of control over actions, concentration on the task, deep but effortless involvement, and a slowing or speeding up of subjective time. During flow, concern for self disappears and there is a loss of consciousness of self. After flow, the sense of self is stronger. The proposed recipe for happiness is to try to create the above flow characteristics.

Although the self may be suspended during flow and perhaps enhanced by flow, this does not necessarily lead to the transpersonal. Similarly, Siddhartha Gautama, before he became the Buddha, mastered the deepest possible levels of concentration meditation, levels far past the self. But the Buddha later explained that these practices only temporally suspend the self and suppress personal defilements. To transcend the self permanently and clean up defilements require a different approach, specifically mindfulness and the eightfold path.

On the other hand, transpersonal and spiritual disciplines have found that the transpersonal can be uncovered when the object dissolves into the subject. This leads to the self as subject and refers back to earlier questions about one's experience of the self as observer and actor.

SELF AS SUBJECT

The mindfulness practices of vipassana include mindful exploration of self as subject (Goldstein, 1993). First one develops a certain degree of concentration and mindfulness while meditating on the contents of the mind, including body sensations, feelings, and thoughts. Later, one turns this focused mindfulness on the behaviors of the mind and on the experience of the subjective self. Seeing into and through the processes one took to be a self is liberating and part of the path to enlightenment.

Within the yogic traditions is the practice of "self-inquiry" taught by Ramana Maharshi (Godman, 1985). The purpose is to try to separate the subjective feelings of "I" and "I am" from the contents of the mind with which they became identified. Since the "I" cannot exist without the object, the "I" disappears, and realization of the transpersonal arises (direct experience of the Self). Part of the practice uses "I" as the object of concentration meditation. Another part of the practice involves a continual search for experiential answers to the questions "Who am I?" and "Where does this I come from?" If a person says he is having trouble doing this practice, then the question is, "What is his direct experience of this self which is having trouble?" The attention is continually directed back toward the "I."

The nondual consciousness that is found through self as subject, among other ways, is professed in the yoga of advaita-vedanta ("nondual end of the vedas," where the vedas are the earliest sacred works of Hinduism and yoga). A good example of how the nondual transcends dichotomies like theistic/nontheistic can be found in the teachings of European Jean Klein (e.g., 1990) and Indian Sri Nisargadatta Maharaj (e.g., Dunn, 1990; Frydman, 1985). Both men were powerful teachers of advaita-vedanta, and their recorded discussions can move those ready to hear. But Maharaj describes the nondual state in terms of God and how we become one with God, which was always true. While Klein almost never makes reference to God or spirituality. He speaks only of consciousness; nothing exists outside of consciousness.

The self, of course, usually does not like the idea that there is no real, separate entity of self. This idea is frightening and threatening. On the other hand, the self often likes the idea of becoming one with the big Self or God. But relative to the nondual, no-self and Universal Self are again like two sides of the same coin. So, up to a point, people can choose the cosmology that speaks to them.

UNIVERSAL PRACTICES

When I surveyed the major psychospiritual disciplines from around the world, Western and Eastern, I found a wide variety of moderately incompatible philosophies, cosmologies, and religions; but when I looked at the psychospiritual practices, I found consensus. That is, if the question is what to do, as opposed to what to believe or think, in order to uncover the transpersonal, then there is agreement. The four, interrelated, universal practices are quieting the mind, increasing awareness, reducing attachments, and opening the heart. This universal path is described briefly next, and elsewhere in more detail with related topics (Mikulas, 1987).

In addition to the universal practices, the great traditions also emphasize the importance of ordering one's life along moral and practical guidelines. There are the Judeo-Christian commandments and the Buddhist precepts. Two of the eight limbs of yoga are abstention from evil conduct (yama) and cultivation of virtuous conduct (niyama). These various guidelines include abstention from killing, stealing, inappropriate sexual behavior, lying, harmful speech, harmful thoughts, greed, and anything that causes suffering.

In Conjunctive Psychology this ethical/practical foundation is built on, and it is recognized that people usually have to do work on the other levels of being before optimally approaching the transpersonal. They need to do things such as get free from the drug, get finances in order, clean up personal relationships, and get unwanted emotions under control. Dealing with these types of issues facilitates uncovering the transpersonal; not dealing with them leaves obstacles to the transpersonal. Hoping that uncovering the transpersonal will eliminate such problems is unrealistic; rather, it will usually make the problems more evident. The level trap involves an individual and/or helper emphasizing approaches that are primarily transpersonal in nature or goal, when emphasis should be given to the other levels. This is a very common trap and is often accompanied by an arrogance that the transpersonal is somehow better than the other levels. In Conjunctive Psychology, all four levels of being are equally valued, and it is recognized that they can be worked with at the same time.

The beauty of the four universal practices is that they impact all levels of being. They could be called meta-level practices or somatopsychospiritual practices. These are the types of approaches given particular emphasis in Conjunctive Psychology, which stresses the total interconnectedness of all levels of being.

For the person with little interest in things transpersonal or spiritual, these practices can be used to dramatically improve physical and mental health, interpersonal effectiveness, and personal happiness and understanding. For the person on a spiritual journey, the practices describe what to do to optimally follow the path of Christianity, Hinduism, Buddhism, or any of the major spiritual or religious traditions.

The first universal practice is quieting the mind, often accomplished by developing concentration. Quieting the mind relaxes mind and body, and thus reduces stress and undesired emotions. It gives us more control over cognitions and creates space to get some distance and perspective on attachments and personal reality. Unless you quiet the mind, you leave the drunken monkey in charge and all you will know is the contents of your own mind, as selected by the monkey. By quieting the mind, you allow the transpersonal to arise and there is more opportunity for insight knowing. As the Third Chinese Patriarch of Zen said, "Stop talking and thinking and there is nothing you will not be able to know." Quieting the mind is the main approach of many yogis and mystics.

The second universal practice is increasing awareness, discussed throughout this book in terms of mindfulness. Increasing mindfulness can lead to greater awareness of and control of body, feelings, body behaviors, contents of the mind, and behaviors of the mind. When this awareness is turned inward, a person becomes aware of mental factors that facilitate and impair uncovering the transpersonal. Continuing inward, mindfulness leads to enlightenment. The impact of mindfulness relative to all levels of being is a major contribution of Buddhist psychology.

The third universal practice is reducing attachments, discussed earlier relative to the clinging behavior of the mind. Reducing attachments clarifies perception, improves thinking, reduces undesired emotions, and increases happiness. Attachments to the self and other aspects of the personal reality are major obstacles to uncovering the transpersonal. And beyond these are subtler and subtler attachments, such as an attachment to not have attachments. Reducing attachments is emphasized in yoga, Buddhism, and Western psychological therapies.

The fourth universal practice is opening the heart, an approach central to Christianity, Mahayana Buddhism, bhakti yoga, and bhakti Hinduism. Opening the heart increases love, empathy, compassion, and peace of mind. There are two aspects to opening the heart: openness and unconditional acceptance. The first involves cultivating a welcoming openness that allows in people and experiences. There are personal "risks" here of becoming involved or hurt. Love, as an ever-expanding force, gradually incorporates more and more while emotions usually create separations.

The second aspect of opening the heart is cultivating unconditional acceptance for reality as it is, even though you are doing things to alter this reality. Accepting does not mean liking or having no preferences. You accept reality as it is in the current moment and act according to appropriate preferences and likes. Similar to the distinction between contents of the mind and behaviors of the mind is the distinction between what is being accepted and the process of accepting. What is being accepted may be desirable or undesirable by various criteria, but the process of accepting is always desirable. Two major traps are distorting perception so the situation is easier to accept, and accepting, but only conditionally.

In cultivation of acceptance and love of other people, it is useful to distinguish between a person's behavior and the essence of the person. We learn to accept unconditionally and to love the essence of the person, regardless of whether we like or dislike the person's behavior. The same is true with the self; one makes friends with one's self, while simultaneously recognizing the need for change, as in one's behavior.

Lovingkindness meditation is a good way to cultivate accepting and loving others (Salzberg, 1997). First, generate feelings of lovingkindness in yourself by whatever method. Traditionally, this was done through repeating statements such as "May all beings be well, happy, and peaceful." Then meditate on a loved one, perhaps a spouse or pet. Over time, gradually work through a meditation hierarchy of many beings, from loved ones, to friends, to people you feel neutral about, to people you have some negative feelings about, and eventually to people whom you have strong negative feelings toward. The key is to move slowly and always maintain the feelings of lovingkindness. (This is an example of the behavior modification practice of counterconditioning.) There are many variations of lovingkindness meditation.

Forgiveness is also often very helpful (Simon & Simon, 1990). Forgiveness is not forgetting or condoning negative behaviors. It does not mean staying in a situation that is unhealthy. Rather, it is letting go of negative emotions, bad memories, grudges, and attachments that create barriers and/or a desire for others to suffer or be punished. To forgive others heals oneself and frees the others. To err is human, to forgive divine.

The four universal practices are totally interrelated; working with one facilitates the others. Hence, it is advantageous to work with all four simultaneously. However, for a particular person at a particular time, it may be best to stress one or more of the practices. The integrative helper aids the client in finding the best way to conceptualize the practices and incorporate them into the broader change program.

Throughout this book, I have recommended that people keep logs, diaries, and mandalas as a way to objectify what they are doing, track progress, and discover patterns and interrelationships. Relative to personal and transpersonal growth, a journal can be very helpful (Baldwin, 1990; Progoff, 1975; Rainer, 1978). The journal includes reflections, and perhaps drawings, related to what you are observing and learning on the journey. Separate sections might be devoted to meditation, mindfulness, attachments, or dreams. Things that might go into the journal include priorities, lists, fantasies, feelings, concerns, obstacles, sources of joy and wonder, decisions, ideas, quotations, myths and teaching stories, other perspectives, unsent letters, and conversations with others (e.g., fictional beings, your body, or your higher self). Writing things in the journal may result in catharsis, producing a reduction in associated negative emotions (respondent extinction). Reading your own journal, you often find general patterns and themes, such as the language you use in describing yourself, the amount of negative thinking, or self-fulfilling prophecies.

Finally, there is a common sequence that arises during personal/transpersonal growth. First, you are lost in the personal reality; you are "of the world." Then gradually you get free from this illusion, as with the universal practices. At this point, you may feel estranged from your prior life and the activities and people related to it. With further progress, you re-enter your life with clarity, compassion, and humor. But you are no longer lost in it as before. You are said to be "in the world, but not of it," an ideal of Christians, Sufis, and others.

ART OF LIVING

A distinction is made between skills of living and the art of living. Skills of living refers to specific practices and techniques a person can utilize to improve her life, such as behavioral self-control strategies, meditation, and the universal practices. Art of living refers to the person's mental set and attitude toward living, including those that occur while she is developing skills of living. This attitude includes moods, associations, expectations, and intentions.

A primary part of the art of living is interested reflection on your life, actively observing your being with a welcoming openness to discover and learn. This can be facilitated by mandalas, journals, diaries, and logs. The second part of the art of living involves taking responsibility for your life and doing things to improve it, as discussed earlier relative to will.

The third part of the art is having fun, enjoying life and not letting the "seriousness" of the melodrama be overwhelming. It includes seeing the cosmic humor in things and being able to laugh at your self. And it involves not "maturing" into a person who forgets how to play.

The fourth part of the art is making friends with your self. Gradually learn to accept and love your self unconditionally while simultaneously recognizing the need for change in some areas. While on the way to some goal, accept where you are at any time rather than become upset that you have not yet reached the goal.

The fifth part of the art is being in the here and now, as much as possible. Spend less time in memories of the past and fantasies of the future. Choose not to be enslaved by events of the past. Try to live more now, rather than continuing to prepare to live in the future. Animals are good teachers about living in the here and now. Relative to transpersonal awakening, it is not a matter of getting "there," but rather being here; it is not something to occur "then," but rather being here now.

Meditation is a wonderful time to cultivate the art of living. The form of meditation can be relatively simple, such as sitting quietly with eyes closed, observing the breath. Here it is easier to be aware of the dynamics of the mind than when you are involved in the complexities of daily living. During meditation, you can observe inertia and resistance to self-discovery and change, and can watch the generating and falling for excuses. Also, you can be aware of all the aspects of the art of living discussed above, which is also the attitude of meditation.

For example, in the early stages of practice most meditators have many thoughts and reactions about meditation and about their capabilities to meditate.

They will evaluate how well they believe they are doing. They will compare themselves with others or their own previous experiences. They will become dissatisfied with their perceived rate of progress and/or what they are experiencing. They will come up with reasons for why they cannot meditate, why meditation is not right for them, or why this is not the best time in their lives for meditating. Most meditators have approach-avoidance reactions toward meditation and some negative feelings about themselves as competent meditators. Hence, an important part of meditation attitude is making friends with your self, accepting where you are relative to meditation, and not getting upset because you are not somewhere else on the path.

Through meditation practice you become aware of the mental dynamics that hinder you from being friends with your self. After developing this awareness in the relatively simple meditation situation, you gradually become more aware of similar dynamics in more complex situations. Meditation practice is a microcosm of living in general. The same is true of all the parts of the art of living. For example, during meditation, you want to simply be in the here and now, not trying to accomplish something. The practice of meditation should be enjoyed in itself, separate from possible future benefits. Parallel examples are dancing and singing, activities that can be enjoyed in the here and now for their own sake, not in terms of where they might lead, such as across the dance floor or to the end of the song.

Finally, the integrative helper is continually looking for ways to help the client with the art of living, since it applies to almost everything the client does. And many other parts of the art could be added to the few listed above, including some of particular importance to a specific client.

INTEGRATIVE HELPERS

Integrative helpers may or may not be personally involved in transpersonal, spiritual, or religious pursuits, but integrative helpers allow for transpersonal possibilities and value clients' interests and concerns with the transpersonal. Of course, the more the helper is personally involved in transpersonal work, such as the universal practices, the more likely the helper can aid clients similarly involved. A common trap here is for helper and/or client to assume that the path that is right for the helper is right for the client.

In addition to general personal/transpersonal development, there is often a transpersonal component in specific helping domains, such as relationships and dying. When assisting people involved in an intimate relationship, helpers may do communication training, contingency contracting, or work with sexual dysfunctions; but, in addition, the relationship can be approached as a shared journey of personal/ transpersonal growth (Campbell, 1980; Welwood, 1990). The relationship provides rich material and attachments to work with. It provides love, support, sparks, and drama for individual and joint transpersonal or spiritual progress. Often a person's mate is the most knowing and caring teacher.

When helping a dying person, you may need to help the person with pain management, getting practical aspects of life in order, and psychological fears and resistance to death (Kübler-Ross, 1969). In addition, for many people death is a time of transition. The transpersonal helper aids the person in understanding this transition within the person's belief system and helps the person approach death with clarity, calmness, and acceptance (Kapleau, 1989; Levine, 1982). For people not about to die, confronting the inevitability of their own deaths can often be an important part of their spiritual growth. Meditating on death is a traditional Buddhist meditation. The classic Tibetan Book of the Dead is a guidebook to read to dying people to prepare them for what they will encounter after death (Fremantle & Trungpa, 1975; Thurman, 1994). But in another sense, we are dying and being reborn every instant. So this book describes transpersonal domains "between" each instant of consensus reality. A translation of the Tibetan title of the book is "The Great Book of Natural Liberation Through Understanding in the Between."

For one who is a professional helper, there are many issues and potential sources of stress, such as difficult or problematic client behaviors, excessive workload and/or paperwork, economic uncertainty, isolation, and burnout (work-related physical, emotional, and/or mental exhaustion). In addition, for the professional helper who is personally involved in transpersonal work, the helping situation is a vehicle for such work (Brandon, 1976; Dass & Gorman, 1985). While helping and serving others, how do you keep from getting lost in or burned out by their suffering and melodramas? How do you keep a clear mind and open heart? How do you avoid power and ego traps and keep from getting caught in an exaggerated view of yourself as helper? When are you really helping, as opposed to pushing your own view or unconsciously succumbing to social/political pressures? And in the midst of all of this, how do you maintain a sense of humor and compassion for yourself and others? The transpersonally oriented integrative helper rejoices at the richness of opportunities for uncovering the transpersonal level of being.

This completes discussion of the four levels of being. In the last chapter, attention will be given to integration and themes across levels.

SUMMARY

The personal-level self comes and goes. For example, it may disappear when a person is very absorbed in some object or action, such as during peak performance or flow experience. It is also possible to experientially move through the self into the transpersonal, as in exploring the self as subject, vipassana meditation, or psychodynamic depth approaches.

Synthesizing all the world's major traditions yields the following for uncovering the transpersonal level of being: order life on moral and practice guidelines, plus the four universal practices of quiet the mind, increase awareness, open the heart, and reduce attachments. Different traditions emphasize different components, but doing all five components satisfies all traditions. All components interact with each other, and all have impact on all levels of being.

In addition to the many skills of living mentioned in this book, there is also the art of living, the mental set and attitude one has toward living. Healthy and helpful parts of the art of living include a welcoming openness, interested reflection, being in the here and now, taking responsibility, making friends with oneself, and having fun.

The integrative helper can incorporate some of the universal practices and art of living into individualized therapies. This will make the therapy package more effective for whatever goals, and simultaneously facilitate uncovering the transpersonal.

AUTHOR'S REFLECTIONS

If you are seriously interested in personal growth and/or uncovering the transpersonal, the four universal practices have great heuristic value. How effective are your current practices, however conceptualized? Part of the answer is how your practices relate to the universal practices. Do they help you quiet your mind, increase awareness, open your heart, or reduce attachments? How balanced and integrated is your overall practice? Again, part of the answer relates to the universal practices. Perhaps you need to do more to open your heart or quiet your mind. Should you join some group, follow some teacher, or take some training? Perhaps. One reason for doing so would be if it provided concrete practical help related to one or more of the universal practices.

Developing skills of living is critical. You must do something that works, not just read and think. The art of living is also important, for everything that you do, including developing skills of living and meditating. The art of living corresponds to the attitude component of meditation practice. This is the component that is least well developed in Western meditation instruction programs, yet the best guidance for meditators, from beginners to advanced practitioners, is often related to meditation attitude.

You may have serious reservations or doubts about the transpersonal. That is fine; there is no problem. You do not have to decide one way or the other, ever! By incorporating the universal practices and art of living into your life, you will improve your life at the biological, behavioral, and personal levels, which is sufficient in itself. In addition, you will allow the transpersonal to gradually arise in a way and at a rate that is appropriate for you. Then you can see for yourself. In fact, this may be a better strategy for uncovering the transpersonal than if you were in quest of it.

THOUGHT QUESTIONS

1. Explain how the subjective self depends on the subject-object duality.
(2.) In what type of clinical situation would the client benefit from exploring the subjective self?
3. Describe an actual or made-up personal experience of flow.
4. For a week, try to practice Buddhist right speech. Avoid vanity and gossip. Try to be helpful and constructive. And for whatever you say or are about

to say, ask yourself if it is true, necessary, and kind. What did you learn from this?

(5.) When seeking to open the heart of a client who has been deeply hurt and thus reticent to allow in people and experiences, how might the integrative helper facilitate the client toward acceptance and forgiveness?

6. For a hypothetical case, describe how you incorporate the general approach of lovingkindness meditation into the overall treatment program.

7. Describe how each of the four universal practices affects each other.

8. What would you add as a fifth universal practice?

9. For a hypothetical case, describe how the universal practices are incorporated into other therapeutic interventions.

10. What things would you put in your own personal journal, and why?

11. Give a practical example of being in the world, but not of it.

(12.) Explain the five parts of the art of living, and how you apply them to yourself.

13. What would you add as a sixth part of the art of living?

14. Why do so many people have more trouble loving and accepting themselves than loving and accepting other people?

(15.) Does making friends with oneself entail recognizing the self as an illusion, or embracing the illusion one takes to be the self, or both?

16. How can a pet teach one about living in the here and now? Give examples.

17. For a hypothetical case, describe how working with the attitude of meditation helps with a specific clinical problem.

18. How can you use your current or future profession to facilitate your own transpersonal uncovering?

PART SIX

ACROSS LEVELS

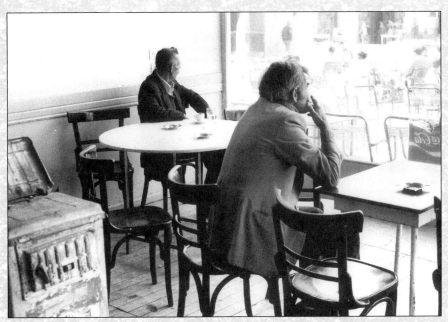

Photo by Benita Mikulas

INTEGRATION AND THEMES

There are two major ways that Conjunctive Psychology differs significantly from NAMAP and from almost all models developed by Western integrative theorists. First is the inclusion of the transpersonal; and second is the greater weight given to biological factors, such as nutrition, breath work, and bodywork. In addition, Conjunctive Psychology encourages investigation of interactions among different levels of being and emphasizes practices that impact several levels, such as the universal practices.

Western psychology became very overspecialized during the second half of the 20th century CE. Research and theories tended to focus on a single level of being, or a subset of a single level. As a result, some of the most surprising findings, and ones that got the most media attention, were interactions across levels, such as how personal-level factors (e.g., self-concept, perception of control) influence biological health.

Therapists who are primarily trained to intervene at one level of being, such as some psychiatrists, behaviorists, humanists, and spiritual helpers, are particularly vulnerable to the level trap, discussed throughout this book. That is, some of the most common and serious errors that helpers make is intervening at the wrong level, such as doing behavior modification when the problem is nutritional, or trying to directly alter self-esteem when behavioral change would be more effective. Because of personal interests and/or client population, an integrative helper might emphasize a particular level of being, but the integrative helper is aware of the significant variables at other levels of being and when a client should be referred to someone else. Integrative helpers cannot be masters of all levels of being, but they can have a broad overview. The major purpose of this book is to stimulate the development of such an overview and to provide key references.

The integrative helper often intervenes at several levels of being simultaneously, switching emphasis depending on the client's needs and therapeutic strategies at different times. But, as a general rule, with many exceptions, it is usually best to deal with biological issues before behavioral issues, behavioral before personal, and personal before transpersonal. For example, it may be best to detoxify a client from a drug, such as alcohol, before doing behavior therapy; help a client learn to control anxiety and anger and develop personal and vocational skills before focusing on self-concept and self-esteem; or facilitate integration of various selves before emphasizing self-transcendence.

This particular sequencing of interventions is common to many theoretical models, including Maslow's hierarchy of needs and the chakra system, the latter described below. Another example is Lane and Schwartz's (1992) "levels of emotional awareness." They suggest five developmental levels, with each level related to the way emotions are processed, type of psychopathology, and appropriate form of intervention. Examples of interventions for the five levels are (1) drugs, relaxation, biofeedback; (2) behavior modification, movement therapy; (3) cognitive therapy, supportive psychotherapy; (4) insight therapy; and (5) existential and insight therapies. Interventions should be based on the appropriate level, proceeding from the lower levels to higher levels. The model is developmental, with successful treatment at one level assumed to move the client to the next level.

Moving from the biological level toward the transpersonal level, it becomes more and more important that helpers be actively involved in working on that level with themselves. Relative to the biological level, it is possible for helpers to give good advice about nutrition and breathing, even though they do not adequately promote their own biological health. But relative to the personal and transpersonal levels, it is much more important that the helpers are actively involved in their own personal/transpersonal development.

Next are considered several themes across levels of being. These are important in their own right and also as an exercise in thinking across levels. Examples of such themes already discussed are the universal practices, objective observation, and mindfulness.

RELAXATION

Relaxation is at one end of a continuum with stress at the other end. Promotion of relaxation at the biological level might involve exercise, bodywork, breath work, or nutritional changes. And most people would profit from some type of body relaxation training, such as muscle relaxation, stretching exercises, or hatha yoga.

At the behavioral level, a major form of relaxation training is quieting the mind, as with concentration meditation. Relaxation, produced by biological and behavioral practices, becomes a reference state for behavioral self-control, such as control of stress, anxiety, or anger. Also at the behavioral level is how a person's lifestyle facilitates or impairs the possibility of relaxation. For example, in the United States, it is common for people to develop a lifestyle that is too complex for biological and psychological health. They try to do too much and do not provide adequate time for relaxing body and mind (Easwaran, 1994). Thus, it is often helpful to work on getting the person's life organized and setting priorities (Lakein, 1973; Winston, 1978). It is also helpful to schedule time for relaxation, play, and being with significant others. Periodic retreats from one's normal life can be rejuvenating and help one gain perspective.

At the personal level, relaxation is often aided by positive thinking, opening the heart, and a sense of humor. One learns how to play the game of life: doing the best one can in a situation and not being vulnerable to winning and losing. Perception of having some degree of control over situations usually reduces stress.

Transpersonal relaxation is based on disidentifying with the self-centered melodrama, as by reducing related attachments. This leads to uncovering a fundamental peace of being. We learn to fight less with reality and more naturally cooperate, an orientation central to Taoism.

HAPPINESS

Purpose and happiness across levels are related since the purpose of many processes is to maximize pleasure, happiness, or peace of mind (Mikulas, 1996b). Purpose at the biological level is largely homeostatic and hedonistic. Homeostasis involves processes for maintaining balance and optimal levels of various biological functions. Hedonistic refers to the tendency to maximize pleasure and minimize pain. Biological bases include endorphins and pleasure and pain areas in the brain. Happiness at the biological level is based on pleasure, balance, and health. There are also the biological correlates of happiness at other levels of being, such as the joy of accomplishment or the bliss of a transcendent experience.

Happiness at the behavioral level involves maximizing reinforcement and minimizing punishment. Reinforcement and punishment include many examples of pleasure and pain, but also much more, particularly social reinforcers. Common sources of happiness at the behavioral level include satisfying and fulfilling relationships, work, and leisure activities (Argyle, 1987; Myers, 1992).

In Conjunctive Psychology, a distinction is made between pleasure and happiness, using the words in specific ways (Mikulas, 1983a). By "pleasure" is meant a short-lived experience due to an enjoyable event or activity. By "happiness" is meant the longer term satisfaction a person has with his life. Pleasure is one possible contributor to happiness, but trying to find happiness by primarily seeking pleasure will seldom work. Pleasure does not last (impermanence), and thus being attached to pleasure often causes suffering (dukkha).

Happiness at the personal level includes four interrelated concerns. First is having a personal reality that is personally satisfying, affectively and conceptually, and that facilitates one's interactions with the world and others. Second is having an integrated sense of self with predominantly positive associations (e.g., positive self-concept, high self-esteem). Third is having the sense that one is capable, to a reasonable extent, of influencing one's self and world in desired directions (e.g., mastery, internal locus of control, high self-efficacy). Personal crises, such as midlife crises, often arise when people have unrealistic goals and expectations for themselves. And fourth is to be in satisfying, supportive, and nurturing relationships with others.

Several sources of happiness, including peace, bliss, and ecstasy, may arise when the transpersonal is uncovered, as in mystical or enlightenment experiences. Some Neo-Platonic philosophers (e.g., John Norris) suggest that contemplative love of God is the source of greatest happiness. And in yoga, a form of bliss as unqualified innate delight (sahaja-ananda) is a property of the absolute ground. Most important for helping is the peace of mind that arises when one disengages from the melodrama of the personal reality, reduces related attachments, opens the heart, and cultivates unconditional acceptance of reality (Keyes, 1975; Watts, 1940). Peace of mind differs from happiness and pleasure, as described above, in that it is less affected by the specifics of situations, has greater equanimity (appreciating and enjoying all things equally), and is potentially longer lasting. Peace of mind is a fundamental result and facilitator of transpersonal development.

DEVELOPMENT OF SELF

In Western psychology's quest to be a science, it chose physics as the model of science to emulate. But, as argued by Irish psychologist Michael Nolan, biology probably would have been a better model. This is particularly true in the area of development.

The development of the self corresponds, to some extent, to the levels of being. A person begins life with no sense of self, the prepersonal stage of development. Then, as the self comes into being, it begins focus on the biological level and gradually moves toward the transpersonal.

The first sense of self is equated with the body. The body is somehow different from other things I perceive: I have more direct control over the body and things that happen to the body produce different sensations from things that happen to other objects. I am the body; the skin separates me from not me. Eventually, possessions may be added to the self. I am my body plus my stuff.

In later stages of development, the body will become part of the self and/or the vehicle the self inhabits. This is particularly true when we watch the body change over time while assuming a constant self in the middle of this change. To the extent that a person is attached to certain properties of the body, perhaps as part of the self, he is particularly vulnerable to what happens to the body. If his self-concept and self-esteem are heavily based on his youthful appearance and strength, psychological suffering (dukkha) is inevitable.

After identification of self with the biological level, development adds in the behavioral level. I am what I do. When answering the question "Who am I?" common responses from most people include personal, social, and vocational roles: I am a Girl Scout and a piano player. I am a mother and a bank president.

Again, the self often includes some of the person's possessions. Many people's sense of self is heavily influenced by things, such as their car or house. Burglary victims often feel personally violated, sometimes raped. And trauma often results from loss of possessions due to natural disasters or when elderly people are put in institutions.

As development moves to include the personal level, a person develops a sense of a self that is a constant entity, separate from body and behaviors. This self, described in detail earlier, is the perceiver of perceptions, willful agent of behaviors, and central character in memories and fantasies. In response to the question "Who am I?" a person might include, "I am the one answering the question."

By now, the person is fully immersed in the personal stage of development. In the United States, important issues for teenagers include identity, relationships with parents, independence, popularity, biological changes, sex, drugs, and suicide. Later, other issues come into play, such as vocation and marriage. As traumatic and melodramatic as many of these issues are for many people, this stage of development cannot be bypassed and should not be devalued. From many perspectives, such as some Hindu and Buddhist cosmologies, the personal stage of development is the reason for incarnation in human form and the optimal opportunity for enlightenment.

Most people will stay stuck in the personal stage of development, but for some others, development will continue and include the transpersonal level. Transpersonal development is described in detail earlier and often includes an intermediate stage where the self is identified with the witness. In response to the question, "Who am I?" the answer might include, "I am the observer of my mind and body."

For many Western and Eastern theorists, uncovering the transpersonal is the final and ultimate stage of development. This is not true in Conjunctive Psychology, where the primary goal is the synthesis and integration of all four levels of being.

CHAKRAS

A particularly heuristic model is the Indian yogic chakra system (Radha, 1978; Rama et al., 1976). A chakra ("wheel") is a center of interaction of body, energy, mind, and consciousness. How "real" chakras are is definitional, debatable, and not important here. The number of chakras varies across systems, from three to more than 20. Here we consider the most popular seven-chakra system. Contemporary interpretations of chakras include seeing them as centers of motivation and attachments, as described below (Dass, 1974; Keyes, 1975).

First is the anal chakra, located near the base of the spine. It is involved with individual survival, security, fear, worry, and paranoia. Second is the genital chakra, located near the genital region. It is involved with survival of the species, sex and lust, and sensory pleasure and pain. Freud was basically a genital chakra theorist. Also applicable are complexity theories and operant learning. A powerful dynamic here is the avoidance of boredom, an important, inadequately researched process, which is having increasing widespread effects in the United States (Mikulas & Vodanovich, 1993).

Third is the navel chakra, located near the spine at the level of the navel. It is involved with power, domination and submission, energy, prestige, pride, gain and loss, success and failure, and praise and blame. Adler was primarily a navel chakra theorist. Also applicable are aspects of assertiveness training and ego psychology.

Fourth is the heart chakra, located between the breasts and near the spine. It is involved with love, compassion, empathy, and generosity, and helps integrate the lower and higher chakras. Aspects of the works of Rogers and Fromm apply here, as do Christianity, Mahayana Buddhism, Bhakti Hinduism, and Bhakti yoga.

Fifth is the throat chakra, located near the thyroid gland. It is involved with receptivity, ability to receive grace and nurturance, surrender, trust, and creativity. Applicable here are aspects of Jung's approach, art and music as devotion, dream analysis, and using concepts to alter the personal reality.

Sixth is the third eye chakra, located between the eyes and just above the eyebrows, in front of the pineal gland. It is involved with insight knowing, intuition, introspection, and the integration of different forms of consciousness, such as from the two brain hemispheres. The Buddha's mindfulness practices apply here.

Seventh is the crown chakra, located at the top of the head. This is the domain of enlightenment and is often illustrated in art by a halo over the head.

The chakra system can be mapped into the four levels of being and used as a way to categorize states of consciousness and psychological problems (e.g., Nelson, 1994; Rama et al., 1976). Relative to development, it is generally held that movement is up through the chakras. This movement is not simple or linear. For example, there is often regression, or one may be primarily functioning from one chakra in some domains and from another chakra in different domains.

As mentioned earlier, relative to the clinging behavior of the mind, chakras are a useful way to categorize attachments. Most people, most of the time, are motivated by attachments related to the first three chakras: security, sensation, and power. Categorizing attachments, as with these three labels, can help in noticing attachments and seeing interrelationships among attachments. In personal and transpersonal growth, a person must first deal with the attachments related to the first three chakras before she can optimally move into the higher chakras. This, of course, is a basic theme of Conjunctive Psychology.

The chakra system is the basis for a model of developmental stages that groups often go through, such as a therapy group or personal growth group (Gilchrist & Mikulas, 1993). The heuristic value of this model is that it specifies the basic dynamic issues and leader interventions for each stage, as well as the relationship of individual development to group process. For example, when the group is at the first stage of development (security), typical dynamics include insecurity, dependency, superficiality, and uninvolvement. Leader actions include establishing rapport, promoting comfort and acceptance, diverting hostility, and providing reassurance. When the group is at the third stage (power), typical dynamics include emotional responses to group issues, manipulative behavior, and dominance and submission. Leader actions include regulating conflict, ensuring closure on each conflict, and facilitating self-understanding and insight.

Earlier, when surveying the biological level, the idea of a life force was discussed. In hatha yoga and tantrism, a female form of the energy is kundalini, which rests at the base of the spine (Scott, 1983; White, 1979). Among other activities, kundalini travels up and down through the chakras, to the extent the chakras are open. Kundalini energizes, balances, and purifies the chakras. When kundalini energizes a chakra or encounters resistance in a chakra, images and feelings related to the theme of the chakra might be elicited. Chakras can be opened in many ways, such as the universal practices. The earlier discussion includes biological and psychological problems that may result from intentional or accidental arousing of kundalini.

The chakra system plus kundalini, like Conjunctive Psychology, cuts across all levels of being and suggests interrelationships between levels. For research purposes, the chakra/kundalini system makes specific predictions about biological correlates of psychological and spiritual phenomena. For Conjunctive Psychology, the chakra system adds to knowledge of developmental sequences and provides a useful category scheme for motivation and attachments.

SUMMARY

Relaxation at the biological level might involve exercise, yoga, breath work, or muscle relaxation. Relaxation at the behavioral level might involve self-control of stress and negative emotions, quieting the mind, or changes in lifestyle. Relaxation at the personal level might involve positive thinking, opening the heart, or cultivating humor. And relaxation at the transpersonal level is related to peace of mind and equanimity.

Happiness at the biological level is based on maximizing pleasure, health, and balance. Happiness at the behavioral level involves maximizing reinforcement and developing a satisfying and fulfilling life. Happiness at the personal level is based on a satisfying and effective personal reality, an integrated self, positive self-concept and high self-esteem, a sense of personal control such as high self-efficacy, and relationships with others that are satisfying, supportive, and nurturing. Happiness at the transpersonal level involves peace of mind, equanimity, rapture, and perhaps bliss or ecstasy.

To a certain extent, development of the self moves across the levels of being, from biological to transpersonal. Each step of development includes the previous, but adds more. A common developmental sequence to the answer to "Who am I?" is: biological, biological plus behavioral, biological plus behavioral plus personal, and those three plus transpersonal.

A chakra is a center of interaction of body, energy, mind, and consciousness. The energy kundalini travels up and down through the chakras, energizing, balancing, and purifying them. This sometimes elicits various biological and psychological experiences. The chakras can be seen as centers of motivation and thus a way to categorize attachments. Many things can be mapped into the chakras, such as personality theories, forms of therapy, psychological problems, and states of consciousness. Development of individuals and some groups tends to correspond to the chakras.

Integrative helpers realize the potential importance of all four levels of being for an optimal change program. Intervention can occur at several levels simultaneously, perhaps involving more than one helper. But the sequencing of the interventions is logically based on factors such as severity of problems, interactions among variables related to various problems or areas of potential growth, the client's needs and desires, the client's motivation and readiness to hear, and the client's state of development in different areas.

The integrative helper may specialize in various ways but always appreciates the importance of maintaining a broad integrated view. The integrative helper does not have all the answers but has learned some of the questions to ask and is open to new ideas from the world's knowledge.

AUTHOR'S REFLECTIONS

I spend a lot of time marveling. One source of marvel is my personal library of books and articles related to the four levels of being. This is an extraordinary collection of information from around the world. In terms of breadth of information on these topics, in one language, my library probably greatly surpasses any library in existence just a few decades ago—the availability of Eastern works in English being a major factor, my past opportunities for international travel and living being another. Of course, now there are probably hundreds of libraries at least as broad in these areas as mine and soon there will be thousands of such libraries, paper and electronic.

The point is that this is an extraordinary time in history for people interested in developing comprehensive and integrated models of psychology and other counseling professions. I have tried to provide a readable overview of basic issues and dynamics. I am most confident that I have included key references for the topics. My major goal for the book is to stimulate thinking. In addition to the reviews of existing knowledge, the book contains considerable "original" material, some of which I hope proves to be heuristic. Conjunctive Psychology is basically an approach that draws from all the world's knowledge and includes all four levels of being and their interactions, however conceptualized. Anyone who agrees with this orientation can be a Conjunctive Psychologist, in addition to other things. There are no dues.

Let us move ahead into much more powerful models, unfettered by past theories and the politics of knowledge. Let us reduce suffering and ignorance, and increase health, love, understanding, wisdom, and awakening.

THOUGHT QUESTIONS

1. For a hypothetical case, give an example of intervening at several levels of being simultaneously.
2. Outline the components of a practical program, for lay community people, entitled "How to find happiness."
(3.) How is it possible to pursue happiness without at least forming an attachment to the notion of happiness?
4. Why might biology be a better model than physics for creating a scientific view of development?
5. Describe your own development as it relates to the four levels of being and the seven chakras.
6. What are the implications of Freud being primarily a genital chakra theorist?

7. Alfred Adler was a sickly child, in rivalry with an athletic older brother. He was short; Freud called him a "pigmy." He was a socialist influenced by Marx and concerned with social issues. His wife was a strong woman and a militant socialist. How does all this relate to Adler's personality theory being primarily third chakra? What are the implications for personality theories in general?

8. How did the heart, an organ that pumps blood, become associated with love (e.g., valentines, "heart-broken")?

9. As a helper at a nursing home, what do you tell relatives of future patients about the role of possessions?

10. For a therapy group, what would be some of the main group issues when the group is at stage four and stage five?

(11.) How might the integrative helper attempt rapprochement between NAMAP and Conjunctive Psychology?

(12.) How do you plan to incorporate theories and ideas from this book into your personal life and your profession?

13. Listing the four levels of being sequentially has some advantages, such as correlations with development and sequencing of interventions. But it can also be misleading. It might suggest that one level is better or higher than another, or it might suggest that some levels are closer to each other. Perhaps a better model is the Conjunctive Pyramid: four triangular faces, where all sides are equal and all corresponding angles are equal. Here, each face (or each corner) corresponds to one of the levels of being. Discuss the advantages and uses of the pyramid. What do different points on or in the pyramid correspond to? What would be the nature of a pyramidal assessment of a person? How does the self relate to the pyramid? Is there some optimal point on or in the pyramid for the self to be?

References

Adams, J. L. (1986). *Conceptual blockbusting* (3rd ed.). Reading, MA: Addison-Wesley.

Ader, R., & Cohen, N. (1993). Psychoneuroimmunology: Conditioning and stress. *Annual Review of Psychology, 44,* 53–85.

Ader, R., Felter, D. L., & Cohen, N. (Eds.). (1991). *Psychoneuroimmunology* (2nd ed.). San Diego, CA: Academic Press.

Ackerman, D. (1990). *A natural history of the senses.* New York: Random House.

Alberti, R. E., & Emmons, M. L. (1975). *Stand up, speak out, talk back.* New York: Pocket Books.

Alberti, R. E., & Emmons, M. L. (1995). *Your perfect right* (7th ed.). San Luis Obispo, CA: Impact Publishers.

Alexander, C. N., & Langer, E. J. (Eds.). (1990). *Higher stages of human development.* New York: Oxford University Press.

Almaas, A. H. (1986). *Essence.* York Beach, ME: Samuel Weiser.

Anderson, C. A. (1989). Temperature and aggression: Ubiquitous effects of heat on occurrence of human violence. *Psychological Bulletin, 106,* 74–99.

Anderson, J. R. (2000). *Learning and memory* (2nd ed.). New York: Wiley.

Andrews, J. (1991). *The active self in psychotherapy.* Boston: Allyn & Bacon.

Argyle, M. (1987). *The psychology of happiness.* London: Methuen.

Arkowitz, H., & Messer, S. B. (Eds.). (1984). *Psychoanalytic therapy and behavior therapy.* New York: Plenum Press.

Assagioli, R. (1965). *Psychosynthesis.* New York: Penguin Books.

Assagioli, R. (1973). *The act of will.* Baltimore: Penguin Books.

Azrin, N. H., & Nunn, R. G. (1977). *Habit control in a day.* New York: Simon & Schuster.

Baldwin, C. (1990). *Life's companion.* New York: Bantam Books.

Ballentine, R. (1978). *Diet & nutrition.* Honesdale, PA: Himalayan International Institute.

Bandura, A. (1997). *Self-efficacy.* New York: W. H. Freeman.

Bankoff, E. A., & Howard, K. I. (1992). The social network of the psychotherapy patient and effective psychotherapeutic process. *Journal of Psychotherapy Integration, 2,* 273–294.

Barker, L. M. (2001). *Learning and behavior* (3rd ed.). Upper Saddle River, NJ: Prentice-Hall.

Baron, R. A. (1987). Effects of negative ions on interpersonal attraction: Evidence for intensification. *Journal of Personality and Social Psychology, 52,* 547–55.

Baron, R. A., & Bronfen, M. I. (1994). A whiff of reality: Empirical evidence concerning the effects of pleasant fragrances on work-related behaviors. *Journal of Applied Social Psychology, 24,* 1179–1203.

Baron, R. A., Rea, M. S., & Daniels, S. G. (1992). Effects of indoor lighting (illuminance and spectral distribution) on the performance of cognitive tasks and interpersonal behaviors: The potential mediating role of positive affect. *Motivation and Emotion, 16,* 1–33.

Baron, R. A., Russell, G. W., & Arms, R. L. (1985). Negative ions and behavior: Impact on mood, memory, and aggression among Type A and Type B persons. *Journal of Personality and Social Psychology, 48,* 746–754.

Batchelor, S. (2000). *Verses from the center.* New York: Riverhead Books.

Beahrs, J. (1982). *Unity and multiplicity.* New York: Brunner/Mazel.

Bear, S., Wabun, W., & Mulligan, C. (1991). *Dancing with the wheel.* New York: Simon & Schuster.

Beck, A. T. (1976). *Cognitive therapy and the emotional disorders.* New York: International Universities Press.

Becker, R. O. (1990). *Cross currents.* New York: Putnam.

Becker, W. C. (1971). *Parents are teachers.* Champaign, IL: Research Press.

Beckson, M., & Cummings, J. L. (1992). Psychosis in basal ganglia disorders. *Neuropsychiatry, Neuropsychology, and Behavioral Neurology, 5,* 126–131.

Bednar, R. L., Bednar, M., Wells, G., & Peterson, S. R. (1989). *Self-esteem: Paradoxes and innovations in clinical therapy and practice.* Washington, DC: American Psychological Association.

Belar, C. D., & Deardorff, W. W. (1995). *Clinical health psychology in medical settings.* Washington, DC: American Psychological Association.

Bellack, A. S., & Hersen, M. (Eds.). (1998). *Behavioral assessment* (4th ed.). Boston: Allyn & Bacon.

Bergin, A. E. (1991). Values and religious issues in psychotherapy and mental health. *American Psychologist, 46,* 394–403.

Bernstein, D. A., & Borkovec, T. D. (1973). *Progressive relaxation training: A manual for the helping professions.* Champaign, IL: Research Press.

Bernstein, D. A., Borkovec, T. O., & Hazlett-Stevens, H. (2000). *New directions in progressive relaxation training.* Westport, CN: Praeger. (Updated version of Bernstein & Borkovec, 1973)

Bigler, E. D., Yeo, R. A., & Turkheimer, E. (Eds.). (1989). *Neuropsychological function and brain imaging.* New York: Plenum Press.

Biner, P. M. (1991). Effects of lighting-induced arousal on the magnitude of goal valence. *Personality and Social Psychology Bulletin, 17,* 219–226.

Birren, F. (1978). *Color and human response.* New York: Van Nostrand Reinhold.

Blanchard, E. B. (Ed.). (1992). Special issue on behavioral medicine. *Journal of Consulting and Clinical Psychology, 60.*

Block, N., Flanagan, O., & Güzeldere, G. (Eds.). (1997). *The nature of consciousness.* Cambridge, MA: MIT Press.

Bly, R. (1990). *Iron John.* Reading, MA: Addison-Wesley.

Bodian, S. (1999). *Meditation for dummies.* Foster City, CA: IDG Books.

Bohart, A. C., & Wugalter, S. (1991). Change in experiential knowing as a common dimension in psychotherapy. *Journal of Integrative and Eclectic Psychotherapy, 10,* 14–37.

Boice, R. (1983). Observational skills. *Psychological Bulletin, 93,* 3–29.

Bonny, H. L., & Savary, L. M. (1990). *Music and your mind.* Barrytown, NY: Station Hill Press.

Boorstein, S. (Ed.). (1996). *Transpersonal psychotherapy* (2nd ed.). Albany: State University of New York Press.

Boorstein, S. (1997). *Clinical studies in transpersonal psychotherapy.* Albany: State University of New York Press.

Boucouvalas, M. (1999). Following the movement: From transpersonal psychology to a multi-disciplinary transpersonal orientation. *Journal of Transpersonal Psychology, 31,* 27–39.

Bourne, E. J. (1995). *The anxiety & phobia workbook* (2nd ed.). Oakland, CA: New Harbinger.

Bowlby, J. (1984). *Attachment and loss: Vol. 1. Attachments* (Rev. ed.). New York: Basic Books.

Bragdon, E. (1990). *The call of spiritual emergency.* New York: Harper & Row.

Branden, N. (1969). *The psychology of self-esteem.* Los Angeles: Nash Publishing.

Brandon, D. (1976). *Zen in the art of helping.* London: Routledge & Kegan Paul.

Braud, W., & Anderson, R. (1998). *Transpersonal research methods for the social sciences.* Thousand Oaks, CA: Sage.

Braun, B. G. (Ed.). (1986). *Treatment of multiple personality disorder.* Washington, DC: American Psychiatric Press.

Brazier, D. (1995). *Zen therapy.* New York: Wiley.

Brewin, C. R. (1996). Theoretical foundations of cognitive-behavioral therapy for anxiety and depression. *Annual Review of Psychology, 47,* 33–57.

Brinthaupt, R. P., & Lipka, R. P. (Eds.). (1992). *The self: Definitional and methodological issues.* Albany: State University of New York Press.

Brockner, J. (1988). *Self-esteem at work.* Lexington, MA: Lexington Books.

Broughton, R. (1975). Biorhythmic variations in consciousness and psychological functions. *Canadian Psychological Review, 16,* 217–239.

Brown, E. F. (1975). *Bibliotherapy and its widening applications.* Metuchen, NJ: Scarecrow Press.

Brown, F. A. Jr., & Chow, C. S. (1973). Interorganismic and environmental influences through extremely weak electromagnetic fields. *Biological Bulletin, 144,* 437–461.

Bruner, J. S., & Postman, L. (1949). On the perception of incongruity: A paradigm. *Journal of Personality, 49,* 206–223.

Brush, F. R., & Levine, E. (Eds.). (1989). *Psychoendocrinology.* San Diego: Academic Press.

Buber, M. (1923). *I and Thou.* (W. Kaufmann, Trans., 1970). New York: Charles Scribner's Sons.

Buchanan, C. M., Eccles, J. S., & Becker, J. B. (1992). Are adolescents the victims of raging hormones: Evidence for activational effects of hormones on moods and behavior at adolescence. *Psychological Bulletin, 111,* 62–107.

Buck, R. (1988). *Human motivation and emotion* (2nd ed.). New York: Wiley.

Buddhadasa Bhikkhu (1992). *Paticcasamuppada: Practical dependent origination.* Nonthaburi, Thailand: Vuddhidhamma Fund.

Buddhadasa Bhikkhu (1997). Mindfulness with breathing (Rev. ed.). Boston: Wisdom Publications.

Buddhaghosa, B. (1975). *The path of purification (Visuddhimagga)* (B. Nanamoli, Trans.) Kandy, Sri Lanka: Buddhist Publication Society.

Burkitt, I. (1991). *Social selves.* London: Sage.

Burns, J. E. (1990). Contemporary models of consciousness: Part I. *Journal of Mind and Behavior, 11,* 153–172.

Burton, D. (1986). *The American Cancer Society's "Freshstart": 21 days to stop smoking.* New York: Pocket Books.

Buss, A. H. (1980). *Self-consciousness and social anxiety.* San Francisco: W. H. Freeman.

Cambell, D. E., & Beets, J. L. (1978). Lunacy and the moon. *Psychological Bulletin, 85,* 1123–1129.

Campbell, J. (1972). *Myths to live by.* New York: Viking Penguin.

Campbell, J. (1986). *Winston Churchill's afternoon nap.* New York: Simon & Schuster.

Campbell, J., & Moyers, B. (1988). *The power of myth.* New York: Doubleday.

Campbell, S. M. (1980). *The couple's journey.* San Luis Obispo, CA: Impact Publishers.

Canada, E. R. (1988). Spirituality, religious diversity, and social work practice. *Journal of Contemporary Social Work, 69,* 238–247.

Caplan, P. J. (1995). *They say you're crazy.* Reading, MA: Addison-Wesley.

Carnegie, D. (1948). *How to stop worrying and start living.* New York: Simon & Schuster.

Carrington, P. (1978). *Freedom in meditation.* Garden City, New York: Anchor Books.

Castaneda, C. (1998). *Magical passes.* New York: HarperCollins.

Catalano, E. M. (1990). *Getting to sleep.* Oakland, CA: New Harbinger.

Cautela, J. R. (1993). Insight in behavior therapy. *Journal of Behavior Therapy & Experimental Psychiatry, 24,* 155–159.

Cautela, J. R., & Groden, J. (1978). *Relaxation: A comprehensive manual for adults, children, and children with special needs.* Champaign, IL: Research Press.

Cautela, J. R., & Kearney, A. J. (1986). *The covert conditioning handbook.* New York: Springer.

Centi, P. J. (1981). *Up with the positive, out with the negative.* Englewood Cliffs, NJ: Prentice-Hall.

Chaiken, S., & Stangor, C. (1987). Attitudes and attitude change. In M. R. Rosenzweig & L. W. Porter (Eds.), *Annual Review of Psychology* (Vol. 38). Palo Alto, CA: Annual Reviews.

Chance, P. (1999). *Learning and behavior* (4th ed.). Pacific Grove, CA: Brooks/Cole.

Charry, J. M., & Hawkinshire, F. B. W. V. (1981). Effects of atmospheric electricity on some substrates of disordered social behavior. *Journal of Personality and Social Psychology, 41,* 185–197.

Chia, M. (1983). *Awakening healing energy through the tao.* Santa Fe, NM: Aurora Press.

Clark, J. (1983). *A map of mental states.* London: Routledge & Kegan Paul.

Claxton, G. (1992). *The heart of Buddhism.* London: Aquarian Press.

Coates, T. J., & Thoresen, C. E. (1977). *How to sleep better.* Englewood Cliffs, NJ: Prentice-Hall.

Cohen, C. (1981). Person categories and social perception: Testing some boundaries of the processing effects of prior knowledge. *Journal of Personality and Social Psychology, 40,* 441–452.

Cohen, R. A. (1993). *The neuropsychology of attention.* New York: Plenum Press.

Cormeir, L. S., & Hackney, H. (1987). *The professional helper.* Englewood Cliffs, NJ: Prentice-Hall.

Cornell, J. (1994). *Mandala.* Wheaton, IL: Quest Books.

Cortright, B. (1997). *Psychotherapy and spirit.* Albany: State University of New York Press.

Coward, H. (1985). *Jung and Eastern thought.* Albany: State University of New York Press.

Craighead, L. W., Craighead, W. E., Kazdin, A. E., & Mahoney, M. J. (Eds.). (1994). *Cognitive and behavioral interventions.* Boston: Allyn & Bacon.

Craik, F. I. M., Moroz, T. M., Moscovitch, M., Stuss, D. T., Winocur, G., Tulving, E., & Kapur, S. (1999). In search of the self: A positron emission tomography study. *Psychological Science, 10,* 26–41.

Cross, S. E., & Madson, L. (1997). Models of the self: Self-construals and gender. *Psychological Bulletin, 122,* 5–37.

Csikszentmihalyi, M. (1990). *Flow.* New York: Harper & Row.

Curtis, R. (1992). Self-organizing processes, anxiety, and change. *Journal of Psychotherapy Integration, 2,* 295–319.

Dalgleish, T., & Watts, F. M. (1990). Biases of attention and memory in disorders of anxiety and depression. *Clinical Psychology Review, 10,* 589–604.

Danaher, B. G., & Lichtenstein, E. (1978). *Become an ex-smoker.* Englewood Cliffs, NJ: Prentice-Hall.

Das, S. (1997). *Awakening the Buddha within.* New York: Broadway Books.

Dass, R. (1974). *The only dance there is.* Garden City, New York: Anchor Books.

Dass, R., & Gorman, P. (1985). *How can I help?* New York: Knopf.

Davey, G. C. L. (1989). UCS revaluation and conditioning models of acquired fears. *Behaviour Research & Therapy, 27,* 521–528.

Davey, G. C. L. (1992). Classical conditioning and the acquisition of human fears and phobias: A review and synthesis of the literature. *Advances in Behaviour Research and Therapy, 14,* 29–66.

Davis, J. (1999). *The diamond approach: An introduction to the teachings of A. H. Almaas.* Boston: Shambhala.

de Bono, E. (1970). *Lateral thinking.* New York: Harper & Row.

de Bono, E. (1982). *de Bono's thinking course.* New York: Facts on File Publications.

de Chardin, T. (1959). *The phenomenon of man.* New York: Harper & Row.

De Maria, E. P., & Mikulas, W. L. (1991). Women's awareness of their menstrual cycles. *Journal of Psychology & Human Sexuality, 4,* 71–82.

de Silva, P. (1984). Buddhism and behaviour modification. *Behaviour Research & Therapy, 22,* 661–678.

de Silva, P. (1985). Early Buddhist and modern behavioral strategies for the control of unwanted intrusive cognitions. *Psychological Record, 35,* 437–443.

Deci, E. L. (1980). *The psychology of self-determination.* Lexington, MA: Heath.

Delgado, J. M. R. (1969). *Physical control of the mind.* New York: Harper & Row.

Delmonte, M. M. (1985). Meditation and anxiety reduction: A literature review. *Clinical Psychology Review, 5,* 91–102.

Dember, W. N., & Warm, J. S. (1979). *Psychology of perception* (2nd ed.). New York: Holt, Rinehart and Winston.

Deregowski, J. B. (1980). Perception. In H. C. Triandis & W. Lonner (Eds.), *Handbook of cross-cultural psychology* (Vol. 3). Boston: Allyn & Bacon.

Dobson, K. S., & Craig, K. D. (Eds.). (1996). *Advances in cognitive-behavioral therapy.* Thousand Oaks, CA: Sage.

Dobzhansky, T. (1972). Genetics and the diversity of behavior. *American Psychologist, 27,* 523–530.

Doweiko, H. E. (1999). *Concepts of chemical dependency* (4th ed.). Pacific Grove, CA: Brooks/Cole.

Duck, S. (1998). *Human relationships* (3rd ed.). Thousand Oaks, CA: Sage.

Dunn, B. R., Hartigan, J. A., & Mikulas, W. L. (1999). Concentration and mindfulness meditation: Unique forms of consciousness? *Applied Psychophysiology and Biofeedback, 24,* 147–165.

Dunn, J. (Ed.). (1990). *Seeds of consciousness* (2nd ed.). Durham, NC: Acorn Press.

Dwairy, M., & Van Sickle, T. D. (1996). Western psychotherapy in traditional Arabic societies. *Clinical Psychology Review, 16,* 231–249.

Dworkin, B. R. (1993). *Learning and physiological regulation.* Chicago: University of Chicago Press.

Easwaran, E. (1994). *Take your time.* Tomales, CA: Nilgiri Press.

Eaves, L., Eysenck, H. J., & Martin, N. (1989). *Genes, culture, and personality.* New York: Academic Press.

Eisenberger, R. (1992). Learned industriousness. *Psychological Review, 99,* 248–267.

Eliade, M. (1975). *Patanjali and yoga.* New York: Schocken Books.

Elliott, R., & Greenberg, L. S. (1997). Multiple voices in process—experiential therapy: Dialogues between aspects of the self. *Journal of Psychotherapy Integration, 7,* 225–239.

Ellis, A., & MacLaren, C. (1998). *Rational emotive behavior therapy.* San Luis Obispo, CA: Impact.

Ellwood, R. (1983). *Finding the quiet mind.* Wheaton, IL: Theosophical Publishing House.

Ellwood, R. S. (1999). *Mysticism and religion* (2nd ed.). New York: Seven Bridges Press.

Emmons, R. A. (1999). *The psychology of ultimate concerns: Motivation and spirituality in personality.* New York: Guilford Press.

Enns, J. T. (Ed.). (1990). *The development of attention.* Amsterdam: North-Holland.

Enright, J. B. (1996). Change versus enlightenment. In S. Boorstein (Ed.), *Transpersonal psychotherapy* (2nd ed.). Albany: State University of New York Press.

Epstein, M. (1995). *Thoughts without a thinker.* New York: Basic Books.

Estes, C. P. (1992). *Women who run with wolves.* New York: Ballantine.

Evans, G. W., Hygge, S., & Bullinger, M. (1995). Chronic noise and psychological stress. *Psychological Science, 6,* 333–338.

Farhi, D. (1996). *The breathing book.* New York: Henry Holt.

Farthing, G. W. (1992). *The psychology of consciousness.* Englewood Cliffs, NJ: Prentice-Hall.

Feinstein, D., & Krippner, S. (1988). *Personal mythology.* Los Angeles: Tarcher.

Feldman, C., & Kornfield, J. (Eds.). (1991). *Stories of the spirit, stories of the heart.* New York: HarperCollins.

Ferrucci, P. (1982). *What we may be.* Los Angeles: Tarcher.

Ferster, C. B., & Culbertson, S. (1982). *Behavior principles* (3rd ed.). Englewood Cliffs, NJ: Prentice-Hall.

Festinger, L. (1964). Behavioral support for opinion change. *Public Opinion Quarterly, 28,* 404–417.

Feuerstein, G. (1998). *The yoga tradition.* Prescott, AR: Hohm Press.

Field, T. (1998). Massage therapy effects. *American Psychologist, 53,* 1270–1281.

Field, T., Morrow, C., Valdeon, C., Larson, S., Kuhn, C., & Schanberg, S. (1992). Massage reduces anxiety in child and adolescent psychiatric patients. *Journal of the American Academy of Child Adolescent Psychiatry, 31,* 125–131.

Field, T. M., Schanberg, S. M., Scafidi, F., Bauer, C. R., Vega-Lahr, N., Garcia, R., Nystrom, J., & Kuhn, C. M. (1986). Tactile/kinesthetic stimulation effects of preterm neonates. *Pediatrics, 77,* 654–658.

Fincham, F. D., Fernandes, L. O. L., & Humphreys, K. (1993). *Communicating in relationships.* Champaign, IL: Research Press.

Fincher, S. F. (1991). *Creating mandalas.* Boston: Shambhala.

Fisher, R. (1971). A cartography of the ecstatic and meditative states. *Science, 174,* 897–904.

Flickstein, M. (2001). *Swallowing the river Ganges.* Boston: Wisdom. (Based on Buddhaghosa, 1975).

Foa, E. B., & Wilson, R. (1991). *Stop obsessing.* New York: Bantam.

Foa, E. B., Zinbarg, R., & Rothbaum, B. O. (1992). Uncontrollability and unpredictability in post-traumatic stress disorder: An animal model. *Psychological Bulletin, 112,* 218–238.

Folkins, C. H., & Sime, W. E. (1981). Physical fitness training and mental health. *American Psychologist, 36,* 373–389.

Forgione, A. G., & Bauer, F. M. (1980). *Fearless flying.* Boston: Houghton Mifflin.

Foreyt, J. P., & Rathjen, D. P. (Eds.). (1978). *Cognitive behavior therapy.* New York: Plenum Press.

Försterling, F. (1985). Attributional retraining: A review. *Psychological Bulletin, 98,* 495–512.

Forsyth, J. P., & Eifert, G. H. (1996). Systemic alarms in fear condition I: A reappraisal of what is being conditioned. *Behavior Therapy, 27,* 441–462.

Foster, S., & Little, M. (1992). *The book of the vision quest.* New York: Fireside.

Frawley, D. (1989). *Ayurvedic healing.* Salt Lake City: Passage Press.

Freemantle, F., & Trungpa, C. (1975). *The Tibetan book of the dead.* Berkeley, CA: Shambhala.

Freesoul, J. R. (1986). *Breath of the invisible.* Wheaton, IL: Theosophical Publishing House.

Freeston, M. H., Ladouceur, R., Thibodeau, N., & Gagnon, F. (1991). Cognitive intrusions in a non-clinical population. I. Response style, subjective experience, and appraisal. *Behaviour Research & Therapy, 29,* 589–597.

Fried, R. (1993). *The psychology and physiology of breathing in behavioral medicine, clinical psychology and psychiatry.* New York: Plenum Press.

Fromm, E. Suzuki, D. T., & de Martino, R. (1960). *Zen Buddhism and psychoanalysis.* New York: Harper & Row.

Frydman, M. (Trans.). (1985). *I am that* (3rd ed.). Durham, NC: The Acorn Press.

Gallup, G. (1995). *The Gallup poll: Public opinion 1995.* Wilmington, DE: Scholarly Resources.

Garrett, J. T. & Garrett, M. (1996). *Medicine of the Cherokee.* Santa Fe: Bear & Co.

Gazda, G. M., Asbury, F. R., Balzer, F. J., Childers, W. C., Phelps, R. E., & Walters, R. P. (1999). *Human relations development: A manual for educators* (6th ed.). Boston: Allyn & Bacon.

Gecas, V., & Mortimer, J. T. (1987). Stability and change in the self-concept from adolescence to adulthood. In T. Honess & K. Yardley, (Eds.), *Self and identity: Perspectives across the lifespan.* London: Routledge & Kegan Paul.

Geen, R. G. (1990). *Human aggression.* Pacific Grove, CA: Brooks/Cole.

Geertz, C. (1973). *The interpretation of cultures.* New York: Basic Books.

Gelso, C. J., & Fretz, B. R. (1992). *Counseling psychology.* Fort Worth: Harcourt Brace Jovanovich.

Gendlin, E. T. (1978). *Focusing.* New York: Everest House.

Gergen, K. J. (1971). *The concept of self.* New York: Holt, Rinehart and Winston.

Gergen, K. J. (1991). *The saturated self.* New York: Basic Books.

Gilchrist, R. (1992). Somatic therapy in recovery. *Professional Counselor,* Feb., 49–51.

Gilchrist, R., & Mikulas, W. L. (1993). A chakra-based model of group development. *Journal for Specialists in Group Work, 18,* 141–150.

Giles, M. M., Cogan, D., & Cox, C. (1991). A music and art program to promote emotional health in elementary school children. *Journal of Music Therapy, 28,* 135–148.

Globus, G. G., Maxwell, G., & Savodnik, I. (Eds.). (1976). *Consciousness and the brain.* New York: Plenum Press.

Godman, D. (Ed.). (1985). *Be as you are: The teachings of Sri Ramana Maharshi.* London: Arkana.

Gold, J. R. (1996). *Key concepts in psychotherapy integration.* New York: Plenum Press.

Golden, C. J., Moses, J. A. Jr., Coffman, J. A., Miller, W. R., & Strider, F. D. (1983). *Clinical neuropsychology.* New York: Grune & Stratton.

Goldfried, M. R. (Ed.). (1982). *Converging themes in psychotherapy.* New York: Springer.

Goldstein, A., & Stainback, B. (1987). *Overcoming agoraphobia.* New York: Penguin Books.

Goldstein, A. P., & Higginbotham, H. N. (1991). Relationship-enhancement methods. In F. H. Kanfer & A. P. Goldstein (Eds.), *Helping people change* (4th ed.). New York: Pergamon Press.

Goldstein, J. (1993). *Insight meditation.* Boston: Shambhala.

Goldstein, J., & Kornfield, J. (1987). *Seeking the heart of wisdom.* Boston: Shambhala.

Goldstein, S., & Goldstein, M. (1990). *Managing attention disorders in children.* New York: Wiley.

Goleman, D. (1971). Meditation as meta-therapy: Hypotheses toward a fifth state of consciousness. *Journal of Transpersonal Psychology, 3,* 1–25.

Goleman, D. (1985). *Vital lies, simple truths.* New York: Simon & Schuster.

Goleman, D. (1988). *The meditative mind.* Los Angeles: Tarcher.

Goreczny, A. J. (Ed.). (1995). *Handbook of health and rehabilitation.* New York: Plenum Press.

Gottman, J., Notarius, C., Gonso, J., & Markman, H. (1976). *A couple's guide to communication.* Champaign, IL: Research Press.

Gray, J. (1993). *Men, women, and relationships.* New York: HarperPaperbacks.

Greenberg, G. S., & Horn, W. F. (1991). *Attention deficit hyperactivity disorders.* Champaign, IL: Research Press.

Greenwald, A. G. (1980). The totalitarian ego: Fabrication and revision of personal history. *American Psychologist, 35,* 603–618.

Gregory, R. L. (1966). *Eye and brain.* New York: McGraw-Hill.

Grof, C., & Grof, S. (1990). *The stormy search for the self.* Los Angeles: Tarcher.

Grof, S. (2000). *Psychology of the future.* Albany: State University of New York Press.

Grof, S., & Grof, C. (Eds.). (1989). *Spiritual emergency.* Los Angeles: Tarcher.

Hamachek, D. (1992). *Encounters with the self* (4th ed.). San Diego: Harcourt Brace Jovanovich.

Hamilton, J. C., Greenberg, J., Pyszczynski, T., & Cather, C. (1993). A self-regulatory perspective on psychopathology and psychotherapy. *Journal of Psychotherapy Integration, 3,* 205–248.

Hanh, T. N. (1975). *The miracle of mindfulness.* Boston: Beacon Press.

Hanser, S. B. (1987). *Music therapist's handbook.* St. Louis: W. H. Green.

Hardin, C., & Banaji, M. R. (1993). The influence of language on thought. *Social Cognition, 11,* 277–308.

Harner, M. (1980). *The way of the shaman.* New York: Harper & Row.

Harrington, A. (Ed.). (1997). *The placebo effect.* Boston: Harvard University Press.

Hart, T., Nelson, P. L., & Puhakka, K. (Eds.). (2000). *Transpersonal knowing.* Albany: State University of New York Press.

Hart, W. (1987). *The art of living.* San Francisco: Harper & Row.

Harvey, J. H., & Weary, G. (1981). *Perspectives on attributional processes.* Dubuque, IA: Wm. C. Brown.

Harvey, J. R. (1998). *Total relaxation.* New York: Kodansha.

Hawkins, S. A., & Hastie, R. (1990). Hindsight: Biased judgements of past events after the outcomes are known. *Psychological Bulletin, 107,* 311–327.

Haynes, S. N., & O'Brien, W. H. (2000). *Principles and practice of behavioral assessment.* New York: Kluwer/Plenum.

Heatherton, T. F., & Baumeister, R. F. (1991). Binge eating as escape from self-awareness. *Psychological Bulletin, 110,* 86–108.

Heine, S. J., Lehman, D. R., Markus, H. R., & Kitayama, S. (1999). Is there a universal need for positive self-regard? *Psychological Review, 106,* 766–794.

Hendlin, S. J. (1983). Pernicious oneness. *Journal of Humanistic Psychology, 23,* 61–81.

Hewitt, J. (1982). *The complete relaxation book.* London: Rider.

Higgins, E. T. (1987). Self-discrepancy: A theory relating self and affect. *Psychological Review, 94,* 319–340.

Hinterkopf, E. (1997). *Integrating spirituality into counseling.* Alexander, VA: American Counseling Association.

Ho, D. Y. F. (1985). Cultural values and professional issues in clinical psychology: Implications from the Hong Kong experience. *American Psychologist, 40,* 1212–1218.

Holdstock, L. (1996). Exploring our relatedness without. In M. G. T. Kwee & T. L. Holdstock (Eds.), *Western and Buddhist psychology: Clinical perspectives.* Delft, The Netherlands: Eburon.

Horton, A. M. Jr., & Miller, W. G. (1985). Neuropsychology and behavior therapy. In M. Hersen, R. M. Eisler, & P. M. Miller (Eds.), *Progress in behavior modification* (Vol. 19). Newbury Park, CA: Academic Press.

Houston, J. P. (1991). *Fundamentals of learning and memory* (4th ed.). Fort Worth, TX: Harcourt Brace.

Hoyle, R. H., Kernis, M. H., Leary, M. R., & Baldwin, M. W. (1999). *Selfhood: Identity, esteem, regulation.* Boulder, CO: Westview Press.

Hung, J. H. F., & Rosenthal, T. L. (1978). Therapeutic video playback: A critical review. *Advances in Behaviour Research and Therapy, 1,* 103–135.

Hunt, E., & Agnoli, F. (1991). The Whorfian hypothesis: A cognitive psychology perspective. *Psychological Review, 98,* 377–389.

Hunt, H. T. (1995). *On the nature of consciousness: Cognitive, phenomenological and transpersonal perspectives.* New Haven, CT: Yale University Press.

Ingersoll, R. E. (1997). Teaching a course on counseling and spirituality. *Counselor Education and Supervision, 30,* 224–232.

Ingram, R. E. (1990). Self-focused attention in clinical disorders: Review and a conceptual model. *Psychological Bulletin, 107,* 156–176.

Iyengar, B. K. S. (1987). *Light on pranayama.* New York: Crossroad.

Jacobs, D. H. (1995). Psychiatric drugging: Forty years of pseudo-science, self-interest, and indifference to harm. *Journal of Mind and Behavior, 16,* 421–470.

Jakubowski, P., & Lange, A. J. (1978). *The assertive option.* Champaign, IL: Research Press.

James, W. (1890/1950). *Principles of psychology.* New York: Dover.

Jeffrey, D. B., & Katz, R. C. (1977). *Take it off and keep it off.* Englewood Cliffs, NJ: Prentice-Hall.

Johnson, D. H. (Ed.). (1995). *Bone, breath, & gesture*. Berkeley, CA: North Atlantic Books.

Johnson, D. H., & Grand, I. J. (Eds.). (1998). *The body in psychotherapy: Inquiries in somatic psychology*. Berkeley, CA: North Atlantic Books.

Johnson, D. W. (1993). *Reaching out* (5th ed.). Boston: Allyn & Bacon.

Johnson, W. (2000). *Aligned, relaxed, resilient*. Boston: Shambhala.

Jones, E. E. (1986). Interpreting interpersonal behavior: The effects of expectancies. *Science, 234*, 41–46.

Julien, R. M. (1997). *A primer of drug action* (8th ed.). New York: W. H. Freeman.

Jung, C. G. (1959). *Mandala symbolism*. Princeton, NJ: Princeton University Press.

Jung, C. G. (Ed.). (1964). *Man and his symbols*. New York: Dell.

Jussim, L. (1986). Self-fulfilling prophecies: A theoretical and integrative review. *Psychological Review, 91*, 429–445.

Jwing-Ming, Y. (1989). *The root of Chinese chi-kung*. Jamaica Plain, MA: Yang's Martial Arts Assoc.

Kahn, E. (1985). Heinz Kohut and Carl Rogers: A timely comparison. *American Psychologist, 40*, 893–904.

Kaku, K. T. (Ed.). (2000). *Meditation as health promotion*. Delft, Holland: Eburon.

Kaplan, B. J. (1972). Malnutrition and mental deficiency. *Psychological Bulletin, 78*, 321–334.

Kaplan, H. B. (1986). *Social psychology of self-referent behavior*. New York: Plenum Press.

Kapleau, P. (1989). *The wheel of life and death*. New York: Doubleday.

Kaptchuk, T. J. (1983). *The web that has no weaver: Understanding Chinese medicine*. Chicago: Congdon & Weed.

Karoly, P., & Kanfer, F. H. (Eds.). (1982). *Self-management and behavior change*. New York: Pergamon Press.

Kaufman, B. N. (1977). *To love is to be happy with*. New York: Fawcett Crest.

Kazdin, A. E. (2001). *Behavior modification in applied settings* (6th ed.). Belmont, CA: Wadsworth.

Keefe, F. J., Kopel, S. A., & Gordon, S. B. (1978). *A practical guide to behavioral assessment*. New York: Springer.

Keen, S. (1991). *Fire in the belly*. New York: Bantam.

Keen, S., & Valley-Fox, A. (1989). *Your mythic journey*. Los Angeles: Tarcher.

Kelly, E. W. Jr. (1995). *Spirituality and religion in counseling and psychotherapy*. Alexandria, VA: American Counseling Association.

Kenny, D. A., & DePaulo, B. M. (1993). Do people know how others view them? An empirical and theoretical account. *Psychological Bulletin, 114*, 145–161.

Kepner, J. I. (1987). *Body process*. New York: Gardner Press.

Kety, S. S., Wender, P. H., Jacobsen, B., Ingraham, L. J., Janson, L., Farber, B., & Kinney, D. K. (1994). Mental illness in the biological and adoptive relatives of schizophrenic adoptees. Replication of the Copenhagen Study in the rest of Denmark. *Archives of General Psychiatry, 51*, 442–455.

Keyes, K. (1975). *Handbook to higher consciousness* (5th ed.). Berkeley: Living Love Center.

Kilmartin, C. T. (1994). *The masculine self*. New York: Macmillan.

Kimble, G. A., & Perlmuter, L. C. (1970). The problem of volition. *Psychological Review, 77,* 361–384.

Kinchla, R. A. (1992). Attention. *Annual Review of Psychology, 43,* 711–742.

Kirschmann, G. J., & Kirschmann, J. D. (1996) (4th ed.). *Nutrition almanac.* New York: McGraw-Hill.

Klein, J. (1988). *Who am I?* Longmead, Shaftesbury, Dorset, England: Element Books.

Klein, J. (1990). *Transmission of the flame.* St. Peter Port, Guernsey, CI: Third Millennium Publications.

Knaster, M. (1996). *Discovering the body's wisdom.* New York: Bantam.

Kohut, H. (1971). *The analysis of the self.* New York: International Universities Press.

Kohut, H. (1977). *The restoration of the self.* New York: International Universities Press.

Kornfield, J. (1993). *A path with heart.* New York: Bantam.

Kübler-Ross, E. (1969). *On death and dying.* New York: Macmillan.

Kunda, Z. (1990). The case for motivated forgetting. *Psychological Bulletin, 108,* 480–498.

Kwee, M. G. T. (Ed.). (1990). *Psychotherapy, meditation & health.* London: East-West Publications.

LaBerge, D. L. (1990). Attention. *Psychological Science, 1,* 156–162.

LaBerge, S. (1985). *Lucid dreaming.* New York: Ballantine.

LaBerge, S., & Rheingold, H. (1990). *Exploring the world of lucid dreaming.* New York: Ballantine.

Lad, V. (1985). *Ayurveda* (2nd ed.). Santa Fe: Lotus Press.

Ladouceur, R., & Mercier, P. (1984). Awareness: An understudied cognitive factor in behavior therapy. *Psychological Reports, 54,* 159–178.

Laing, R. D. (1960). *The divided self: An existential study in sanity and madness.* London: Tavistock.

Lajoie, D. H., & Shapiro, S. J. (1992). Definitions of transpersonal psychology: The first twenty-three years. *Journal of Transpersonal Psychology, 24,* 79–98.

Lakein, A. (1973). *How to get control of your time and your life.* New York: Wyden.

Lamberton, L. H., & Minor, L. (1995). *Human relations.* Chicago: Irwin Mirror Press.

Landrine, H. (1992). Clinical implications of cultural differences: The referential versus the indexical self. *Clinical Psychology Review, 12,* 401–413.

Lane, R. D., & Schwartz, G. E. (1992). Levels of emotional awareness: Implications for psychotherapeutic integration. *Journal of Psychotherapy Integration, 2,* 1–18.

Lange, A. J., & Jakubowski, P. (1976). *Responsible assertive behavior.* Champaign, IL: Research Press.

Lapsley, D. K., & Power, F. C. (Eds.). (1988). *Self, ego, and identity: Integrative approaches.* New York: Springer-Verlag.

Lark, S. M. (1995). *The estrogen decision self-help book* (Rev. ed.). Berkeley, CA: Celestial Arts.

Larrick, R. P. (1993). Motivational factors in decision theories: The role of self-protection. *Psychological Bulletin, 113,* 440–450.

Lasure, L. C., & Mikulas, W. L. (1996). Biblical behavior modification. *Behaviour Research & Therapy, 34,* 563–566.

Lavy, E., van den Hout, M., & Arntz, A. (1993). Attentional bias and spider phobia: Conceptual and clinical issues. *Behaviour Research & Therapy, 31,* 17–24.

Lazarick, D. L., Fishbein, S. S., Loiello, M. A., & Howard, G. S. (1988). Practical investigation of volition. *Journal of Counseling Psychology, 35,* 15–26.

Leccese, A. P. (1991). *Drugs and society.* Englewood Cliffs, NJ: Prentice-Hall.

Lefcourt, H. M. (1976). Locus of control and the response to aversive events. *Canadian Psychological Review, 17,* 202–209.

Lefcourt, H. M. (1982). *Locus of control* (2nd ed.). Hillsdale, NJ: Erlbaum.

Leon, M. (1992). The neurobiology of filial learning. *Annual Review of Psychology, 43,* 377–398.

Lesh, T. V. (1970). Zen meditation and the development of empathy in helpers. *Journal of Humanistic Psychology, 10,* 39–74.

LeShan, L. (1974). *How to meditate.* New York: Bantam.

Levant, R. F. (1995). *Masculinity reconstructed.* New York: Dutton.

Levine, S. (1982). *Who dies?* Garden City, NY: Anchor Books.

Levis, D. J. (1989). The case for a return to a two-factor theory of avoidance: The failure of non-fear interpretations. In S. B. Klein & R. R. Mowrer (Eds.), *Contemporary learning theories.* Hillsdale, NJ: Erlbaum.

Lewinsohn, P. M., Munoz, R. F., Youngren, M. A., & Zeiss, A. M. (1992). *Control your depression.* New York: Fireside.

Ley, R. (1999). The modification of breathing behavior. *Behavior Modification, 23,* 441–479.

Li-Repac, D. (1980). Cultural influences on clinical perceptions: A comparison between Caucasian and Chinese American therapists. *Journal of Cross-Cultural Psychology, 11,* 327–342.

Libet, B., Gleason, C. A., Wright, E. W., & Pearl, D. K. (1983). Time of intention to act in relation to onset of cerebral activity (readiness potential). *Brain, 106,* 623–642.

Lieber, A. L. (1978). *The lunar effect: Biological tides and human emotions.* Garden City, NJ: Doubleday.

Lillard, A. (1998). Ethnopsychologies: Cultural variations in theories of mind. *Psychological Bulletin, 123,* 3–32.

Lilly, J. C. (1972). *The center of the cyclone.* New York: Bantam.

Linden, W. (1973). Practicing of meditation by school children and their levels of field dependence-independence, test anxiety, and reading achievement. *Journal of Consulting and Clinical Psychology, 41,* 139–143.

Linehan, M. M. (1988). Perspectives on the interpersonal relationship in behavior therapy. *Journal of Integrative & Eclectic Psychotherapy, 7,* 278–290.

Linville, P. W. (1987). Self-complexity as a cognitive buffer against stress-related illness and depression. *Journal of Personality and Social Psychology, 52,* 633–676.

Lockard, J. S., & Paulhus, D. L. (Eds.). (1988). *Self-deception: An adaptive mechanism?* Englewood Cliffs, NJ: Prentice-Hall

Locke, S., & Colligan, D. (1986). *The healer within.* New York: Dutton.

Loftus, E. F., Miller, D. G., & Burns, H. J. (1978). Semantic integration of verbal information into a visual memory. *Journal of Experimental Psychology: Human Learning and Memory, 4,* 19–31.

Logue, A. W. (1995). *Self-control.* Englewood Cliffs, NJ: Prentice-Hall.

London, P. (1969). *Behavioral control.* New York: Harper & Row.

Love, S. M. (1997). *Dr. Susan Love's hormone book.* New York: Random House.

Lozoff, B. (1989). Nutrition and behavior. *American Psychologist, 44,* 231–236.

Luce, G. G. (1971). *Body time.* New York: Bantam.

Lukoff, D. (1985). The diagnosis of mystical experience with psychotic features. *Journal of Transpersonal Psychology, 17,* 155–181.

Lukoff, D. (1996). Transpersonal psychotherapy with psychotic disorders and spiritual emergencies with psychotic features. In B. W. Scotton, A. B. Chinen, & J. R. Battista (Eds.), *Textbook of transpersonal psychiatry and psychology.* New York: Basic Books.

Lustman, P. J., Griffith, L. S., Clouse, R. E., & Cryer, P. E. (1986). Psychiatric illness in diabetes mellitus. Relationship to symptoms and glucose control. *Journal of Nervous and Mental Disease, 174,* 736–742.

Lykken, D. T., McGue, M., Tellegen, A., & Bouchard, T. J. Jr., (1992). Emergenesis: Genetic traits that may not run in families. *American Psychologist, 47,* 1565–1577.

Lynch, M. D., Noren-Hebeisen, A. A., & Gergen, K. J. (Eds.). (1981). *Self-concept.* Cambridge, MA: Ballinger.

Maag, J. W. (1999). *Behavior management.* San Diego: Singular Publishing Group.

MacDonald, D. A., Friedman, H. L., & Kuentzel, J. G. (1999a). A survey of measures of spiritual and transpersonal constructs: Part one—research update. *Journal of Transpersonal Psychology, 31,* 137–154.

MacDonald, D. A., Kuentzel, J. G., & Friedman, H. L. (1999b). A survey of measures of spiritual and transpersonal constructs: Part two—additional instruments. *Journal of Transpersonal Psychology, 31,* 155–178.

MacDonald, D. A., LeClair, L., Holland, C. J., Alter, A., & Friedman H. L. (1995). A survey of measures of transpersonal constructs. *Journal of Transpersonal Psychology, 27,* 171–235.

MacTurk, R. H., & Morgan, G. A. (Eds.). (1995). *Mastery motivation.* Norwood, NJ: Ablex.

Mager, R. F. (1997). *Goal analysis.* (3rd ed.). Atlanta, GA: Center for Effective Performance.

Mahasi Sayadaw (1978). *The progress of insight.* Kandy, Sri Lanka: Buddhist Publication Society.

Mahasi Sayadaw (1980). *Practical insight meditation.* Kandy, Sri Lanka: Buddhist Publication Society.

Mahoney, M. J. (1991). *Human change processes.* New York: Basic Books.

Mahrer, A. R. (1989). *An integration of psychotherapies.* New York: Human Science Press.

Maier, S. F., Watkins, L. R., & Fleshner, M. (1994). Psychoneuroimmunology: The interface between behavior, brain, and immunity. *American Psychologist, 49,* 1004–1017.

Markus, H. (1990). Unresolved issues of self-representation. *Cognitive Therapy and Research, 14,* 241–253.

Markus, H. R., & Kitayama, S. (1991). Culture and the self: Implications for cognition, emotion, and motivation. *Psychological Review, 98,* 224–253.

Marshall, P. (1989). Attention deficit disorder and allergy: A neurochemical model of the relation between the illnesses. *Psychological Bulletin, 106,* 434–446.

Martin, D. G. (1983). *Counseling and therapy skills.* Prospect Heights, IL: Waveland Press.

Martin, G., & Pear, J. (1999). *Behavior modification* (6ᵗʰ ed.). Upper Saddle River, NJ: Prentice-Hall.

Martin, I., & Levey, A. B. (1978). Evaluative conditioning. *Advances in Behavioural Research and Therapy, 1,* 57–102.

Maslow, A. (1968). *Toward a psychology of being* (Rev. ed.). Princeton, NJ: Van Nostrand.

Maslow, A. (1970). *Religions, values, and peak experiences.* New York: Viking.

Matsumoto, D. (1996). *Culture and psychology.* Pacific Grove, CA: Brooks/Cole.

Maul, G., & Maul, T. (1983). *Beyond limit.* Glenview, IL: Scott, Foresman.

Maxmen, J. S. (1981). *A good night's sleep.* New York: Warner.

May, R. (1969). *Love and will.* New York: Norton.

McCullough, M. E., Hoyt, W. T., Larson, D. B., Koenig, H. G., & Thoresen, C. (2000). Religious involvement and mortality: A meta-analytic review. *Health Psychology, 19,* 211–222.

McGaa, E. (Eagle Man). (1990). *Mother earth spirituality.* San Francisco: HarperCollins.

McGuigan, F. J. (1981). *Calm down.* Englewood Cliffs, NJ: Prentice-Hall.

McLaughlin, M. L., Cody, M. J., & Read, S. J. (Eds.). (1992). *Explaining one's self to others.* Hillsdale, NJ: Erlbaum.

McNally, R. J. (1987). Preparedness and phobias: A review. *Psychological Bulletin, 101,* 283–303.

Meharg, S. S., & Woltersdorf, M. A. (1990). Therapeutic use of videotape self-modeling: A review. *Advances in Behaviour Research and Therapy, 12,* 85–99.

Menzies, R. G., & Clarke, J. C. (1995). The etiology of phobias: A nonassociative account. *Clinical Psychology Review, 15,* 23–48.

Merrell-Wolff, F. (1973). *The philosophy of consciousness without an object.* New York: Julian Press.

Messer, S. C., Morris, T. L., & Gross, A. M. (1990). Hypoglycemia and psychopathology: A methodological review. *Clinical Psychology Review, 10,* 631–648.

Meth, R. L., & Pasick, R. S. (1990). *Men in therapy.* New York: Guilford Press.

Metzner, R. (1989). States of consciousness and transpersonal psychology. In R. Vallee & S. Halling (Eds.), *Existential-phenomenological perspectives in psychology.* New York: Plenum Press.

Metzner, R. (1996). The Buddhist six-worlds model of consciousness and reality. *Journal of Transpersonal Psychology, 28,* 155–166.

Metzner, R. (1998). *The unfolding self.* Novato, CA: Origin Press.

Mikulas, W. L. (1974). *Concepts in learning.* Philadelphia: W. B. Saunders.

Mikulas, W. L. (1978a). *Behavior modification.* New York: Harper & Row.

Mikulas, W. L. (1978b). Four noble truths of Buddhism related to behavior therapy. *Psychological Record, 28,* 59–67.

Mikulas, W. L. (1981). Buddhism and behavior modification. *Psychological Record, 31,* 331–342.

Mikulas, W. L. (1983a). *Skills of living.* Lanham, MD: University Press of America.

Mikulas, W. L. (1983b). Thailand and behavior modification. *Journal of Behavior Therapy and Experimental Psychology, 14,* 93–97.

Mikulas, W. L. (1986). Self-control: Essence and development. *Psychological Record,* *36,* 297–308.

Mikulas, W. L. (1987). *The way beyond.* Wheaton, IL: Theosophical Publishing House.

Mikulas, W. L. (1990). Mindfulness, self-control, and personal growth. In M. G. T. Kwee (Ed.), *Psychotherapy, meditation, & health.* London: East-West Publications.

Mikulas, W. L. (1991). Eastern and Western psychology: Issues and domains for integration. *Journal of Integrative and Eclectic Psychotherapy, 10,* 229–240.

Mikulas, W. L. (1995). Conjunctive Psychology: Issues of integration. *Journal of Psychotherapy Integration, 5,* 331–348.

Mikulas, W. L. (1996a). Sudden onset of subjective dimensionality: A case study. *Perceptual and Motor Skills, 82,* 852–854.

Mikulas, W. L. (1996b). Toward a conjunctive psychology: Happiness and levels of being. In M. G. T. Kwee & T. L. Holdstock (Eds.), *Western and Buddhist psychology.* Delft, Holland: Eburon.

Mikulas, W. L. (2000). Behaviors of the mind, meditation, and health. In K. T. Kaku (Ed.), *Meditation as health promotion.* Delft, Holland: Eburon.

Mikulas, W. L., & Coffman, M. G. (1989). Home-based treatment of children's fear of the dark. In C. E. Schaefer, & J. M. Briesmeister, (Eds.), *Handbook of parent training.* New York: Wiley.

Mikulas, W. L., Coffman, M. G., Dayton, D., Frayne, C., & Maier, P. L. (1985). Behavioral bibliotherapy and games for treating fear of the dark. *Child & Family Behavior Therapy, 7,* 1–7.

Mikulas, W. L., & Vodanovich, S. J. (1993). The essence of boredom. *Psychological Record, 43,* 3–12.

Miller, N. E. (1971). *Neal E. Miller: Selected papers.* Chicago: Aldine Atherton.

Miller, S. M. (1979). Controllability and human stress: Method, evidence, and theory. *Behaviour Research and Therapy, 17,* 287–304.

Miltenberger, R. (2001). *Behavior modification* (2nd ed.). Belmont, CA: Wadsworth.

Mishra, R. S. (1987). *The textbook of yoga psychology.* New York: Julian Press.

Moir, A., & Jessel, D. (1991). *Brain sex.* New York: Carol Publishing.

Moldin, S. O., Reich, T., & Rice, J. P. (1991). Current perspectives on the genetics of unipolar depression. *Behavior Genetics, 21,* 211–242.

Mook, D. G. (1996). *Motivation* (2nd ed.). New York: Norton.

Moran, A. P. (1996). *The psychology of concentration in sports performers.* East Sussex, UK: Psychology Press.

Moray, N. (1969). *Attention.* New York: Academic Press.

Morgan, W. P. (Ed.). (1997). *Physical activity and mental health.* Washington, DC: Taylor & Francis.

Morin, C. M. (1996). *Relief from insomnia.* New York: Doubleday.

Muller, W. (1999). *Sabbath: Restoring the sacred rhythm of rest.* New York: Bantam.

Murphy, M. (1992). *The future of the body.* Los Angeles: Jeremy P. Tarcher.

Murphy, M., & Donovan, S. (1997). *The physical and psychological effects of meditation* (2nd ed.). Sausalito, CA: Institute of Noetic Sciences.

Murphy, M., & White, R. A. (1978). *The psychic side of sports.* Reading, MA: Addison-Wesley.

Murphy, M., & White, R. A. (1995). *In zone.* New York: Penguin Arkana.

Myers, D. G. (1992). *The pursuit of happiness.* New York: William Morrow.

Myers, D. G. (2000). The funds, friends, and faith of happy people. *American Psychologist, 55,* 56–67.

Nadeau, S. E., & Crosson, B. (1995). A guide to the functional imaging of cognitive processes. *Neuropsychiatry, Neuropsychology, and Behavioral Neurology, 8,* 143–162.

Nairn, R. (1999). *Diamond mind.* Boston: Shambhala.

Neath, I. (1998). *Human memory.* Pacific Grove, CA: Brooks/Cole.

Needleman, H. L., Riess, J. A., Tobin, M. J., Biesecker, G. E., & Greenhouse, J. B. (1996). Bone lead levels and delinquent behavior. *Journal of the American Medical Association, 275,* 363–369.

Neimeyer, R. A. (1993). An appraisal of constructivist psychotherapies. *Journal of Consulting and Clinical Psychology, 61,* 221–234.

Nelson, J. E. (1994). *Healing the split* (Rev. ed.). Albany: State University of New York Press.

Nelson, R. J., Badura, L. L., & Goldman, B. D. (1990). Mechanisms of seasonal cycles of behavior. *Annual Review of Psychology, 41,* 81–108.

Norbu, N. (1992). *Dream yoga and the practice of natural light.* Ithaca, NY: Snow Lion.

Norcross, J. C., & Goldfried, M. R. (Eds.). (1992). *Handbook of psychotherapy integration.* New York: Basic Books.

Null, G. (1995). *Nutrition and the mind.* New York: Four Walls Eight Windows.

Nyanaponika Thera. (1962). *The heart of Buddhist meditation.* London: Rider and Co.

Nyanatiloka Mahathera. (1971). *Guide through the abhidhamma-pitaka.* Kandy, Sri Lanka: Buddhist Publication Society.

O'Banion, D. R., & Whaley, D. L. (1981). *Behavior contracting.* New York: Springer.

O'Brien, J., & Kollock, P. (Eds.). (1997). *The production of reality* (2nd ed.). Thousand Oaks, CA: Pine Forge Press.

O'Leary, A. (1990). Stress, emotion, and human immune function. *Psychological Bulletin, 108,* 363–382.

O'Leary, K. D., & Wilson, G. T. (1987). *Behavior therapy* (2nd ed.). Englewoods Cliffs, NJ: Prentice-Hall.

Orenstein, N. S., & Bingham, S. L. (1987). *Food allergies.* New York: Putnam.

Ornstein, R. E. (1986). *The psychology of consciousness* (Rev. ed.). New York: Viking Penguin.

Ortiz, J. M. (1997) *The tao of music.* York Beach, MA: Samuel Weiser.

Pachuta, D. M. (1996). Chinese medicine: The law of five elements. In A. A. Sheikh, & K. S. Sheikh, (Eds.), *Healing east and west.* New York: Wiley.

Paley, V. (1984). *Boys and girls.* Chicago: University of Chicago Press.

Parasuraman, R. (Ed.). (1998). *The attentive brain.* Cambridge, MA: MIT Press.

Patterson, G. R. (1975). *Families* (Rev. ed.). Champaign, IL: Research Press.

Patterson, G. R., & Forgatch, M. (1987). *Parents and adolescents living together.* Eugene, OR: Castalia Publishing.

Pedersen, P. B., Draguns, J. G., Lonner, W. J., & Trimble, J. E. (Eds.). (1996). *Counseling across cultures.* Thousand Oaks, CA: Sage.

Pelletier, K. R. (1977). *Mind as healer, mind as slayer.* New York: Delta.

Pelletier, K. R. (1978). *Toward a science of consciousness.* New York: Delta.

Peterson, C., Maier, S. F., & Seligman, M. E. P. (1993). *Learned helplessness.* New York: Oxford University Press.

Peurifoy, R. Z. (1988). *Anxiety, phobias, & panic.* Citrus Heights, CA: Life Skills.

Phelps, E. J. (1981). *The maids of the north.* New York: Holt.

Pierce, W. D., & Epling, W. F. (1999). *Behavior analysis and learning* (2nd ed.). Englewood Cliffs, NJ: Prentice-Hall.

Poling, A., Gadow, K. D., & Cleary, J. (1991). *Drug therapy for behavior disorders: An introduction.* New York: Pergamon Press.

Ponterotto, J. G., Casas, J. M., Suzuki, L. A., & Alexander, C. M. (Eds.). (1995). *Handbook of multicultural counseling.* Thousand Oaks, CA: Sage.

Prabhavanda, Swami, & Isherwood, C. (1953). *How to know God: The yoga aphorisms of Patanjali.* New York: Mentor.

Prigatano, G. P. (1992). Personality disturbances associated with traumatic brain injury. *Journal of Consulting and Clinical Psychology, 60,* 360–368.

Prochaska, J. O., & DiClemente, C. C. (1984). *The transtheoretical approach.* Homewood, IL: Dow Jones-Irwin.

Progoff, I. (1975). *At a journal workshop.* New York: Dialogue House Library.

Rachman, S. (1997). A cognitive theory of obsessions. *Behaviour Research & Therapy, 35,* 793–802.

Rachman, S., & de Silva, P. (1996). *Panic disorder.* New York: Oxford University Press.

Radha, Swami S. (1978). *Kundalini: Yoga for the West.* Spokane, WA: Timeless Books.

Rahula, W. (1974). *What the Buddha taught* (2nd ed.). New York: Grove Press.

Rainer, T. (1978). *The new diary.* Los Angeles: Tarcher.

Rama, Swami. (1986). *Path of fire and light.* Honesdale, PA: Himalayan International Institute.

Rama, Swami, Ballentine, R., & Ajaya, Swami. (1976). *Yoga and psychotherapy.* Glenview, IL: Himalayan Institute.

Rama, Swami, Ballentine, R., & Hymes, A. (1979). *Science of breath.* Honesdale, PA: Himalayan International Institute.

Rank, O. (1929). *Will therapy and truth and reality.* (J. Taft, Trans., 1945). New York: Knopf.

Rao, S. M., Huber, S. J., & Bornstein, R. A. (1992). Emotional changes with multiple sclerosis and Parkinson's disease. *Journal of Consulting and Clinical Psychology, 60,* 369–378.

Rassin, E., Merckelbach, H., & Muris, P. (2000). Paradoxical and less paradoxical effects of thought suppression: A critical review. *Clinical Psychology Review, 8,* 973–995.

Raz, S., & Raz, N. (1990). Structural brain abnormalities in the major psychoses: A quantitative review of the evidence from computerized imagining. *Psychological Bulletin, 108,* 93–108.

Reese, E. P. (1978). *Human operant behavior* (2nd ed.). Dubuque, IA: Wm. C. Brown.

Reiff, D. W., & Reiff, K. K. L. (1992). *Eating disorders: Nutrition therapy in the recovery process.* Gaithersburg, MD: Aspen.

Renfrew, J. W. (1997). *Aggression and its causes.* New York: Oxford University Press.

Reps, P. (Ed.). (1957). *Zen flesh, Zen bones.* Garden City, New York: Doubleday.

Rescorla, R. A. (1988). Pavlovian conditioning: It's not what you think it is. *American Psychologist, 43,* 151–160.

Rescorla, R. A., & Solomon, R. L. (1967). Two-process learning theory: Relationships between Pavlovian conditioning and instrumental learning. *Psychological Review, 74,* 151–182.

Ring, K. (1976). Mapping the regions of consciousness: A conceptual reformulation. *Journal of Transpersonal Psychology, 8,* 77–88.

Rippere, V. (1983). Nutritional approaches to behavior modification. In M. Hersen, R. M. Eisler, & P. M. Miller (Eds.), *Progress in behavior modification* (Vol. 14). New York: Academic Press.

Ritter, M., & Low, K. G. (1996). Effects of dance/movement therapy: A meta-analysis. *The Arts in Psychotherapy, 23,* 249–260.

Roberts, A. H., Kewman, D. G., Mercier, L., & Hovell, M. (1993). The power of nonspecific effects in health: Implications for psychosocial and biological treatments. *Clinical Psychology Review, 13,* 375–391.

Rogers, C. R. (1951). *Client-centered therapy.* Boston: Houghton Mifflin.

Rogers, C. R. (1961). *On becoming a person.* Boston: Houghton Mifflin.

Rorer, L. G. (1983). "Deep" RET: A reformulation of some psychodynamic explanations of procrastination. *Cognitive Therapy and Research, 7,* 1–10.

Rose, E. M., Westefeld, J. S., & Ansley, T. N. (2001). Spiritual issues in counseling: Clients' beliefs and preferences. *Journal of Counseling Psychology, 48,* 61–71.

Rosen, G. M. (1977). *The relaxation book: an illustrated self-help program.* Englewood Cliffs, NJ: Prentice-Hall.

Rosen, H., & Kuehlwein, K. T. (Eds.). (1996). *Constructing realities.* San Francisco: Jossey-Bass.

Rosen, S. (1979). *Weathering.* New York: M. Evans and Co.

Rosenberg, L. (1999). *Breath by breath.* Boston: Shambhala.

Rosenfarb, I. S. (1992). A behavior analytic interpretation of the therapeutic relationship. *Psychological Record, 42,* 341–354.

Rosenthal, N. E. (1998). *Winter blues.* New York: Guilford.

Rosenthal, R., & Jacobson, L. (1968). *Pygmalion in the classroom: Teacher expectations and pupils' intellectual development.* New York: Holt, Rinehart & Winston.

Rossi, E. R. (1986). Altered states of consciousness in everyday life: The Ultradian rhythms. In B. B. Wolman & M. Ullman (Eds.), *Handbook of states of consciousness.* New York: Van Nostrand Reinhold.

Rothbaum, F., Weisz, J., Pott, M., Miyake, K., & Morelli, G. (2000). Attachment and culture. *American Psychologist, 55,* 1093–1104.

Rotten, J., & Kelly, I. W. (1985). Much ado about the full moon: A meta-analysis of lunar-lunacy research. *Psychological Bulletin, 97,* 286–306.

Rotter, J. B. (1966). Generalized expectancies of internal versus external control of reinforcement. *Psychological Monographs, 80,* whole No. 609.

Rowan, R. (1993). *The transpersonal.* London: Routledge.

Rubin, E. H. (1992). Delusions as part of Alzheimer's disease. The schizophrenia-like psychosis of epilepsy. *Neuropsychiatry, Neuropsychology, and Behavioral Neurology, 5,* 108–113.

Rubin, R. J. (1978). *Using bibliotherapy.* Phoenix: Oryx Press.

Ruitenbeek, H. M. (Ed.). (1972). *Going crazy.* New York: Bantam.

Ryman, D. (1993). *Aromatherapy.* New York: Bantam.

Salmon, P. (2001). Effects of physical exercise on anxiety, depression, and sensitivity to stress: A unifying theory. *Clinical Psychology Review, 21,* 33–61.

Salovey, P., Rothman, B. J., Detweiler, J. B., & Steward W. T. (2000). Emotional states and physical health. *American Psychologist, 55,* 110–121.

Salzberg, S. (1997). *Lovingkindness.* Boston: Shambhala.

Sanchez, V. (1995). *The teaching of Don Carlos.* Santa Fe, NM: Bear & Co.

Sannella, L. (1987). *The kundalini experience.* Lower Lake, CA: Integral Publishing.

Sapolsky, R. M. (1998). *Why zebras don't get ulcers.* New York: W. H. Freeman.

Sappington, A. A. (1990). Recent psychological approaches to the free-will versus determinism issue. *Psychological Bulletin, 108,* 19–29.

Sarafino, E. P. (1998). *Health psychology* (3rd ed.) New York: Wiley.

Savitripriya, Swami. (1991). *Psychology of mystical awakening.* Sunnyvale, CA: New Life Books.

Schacter, D. L. (1996). *Searching for memory.* New York: Basic Books.

Schacter, D. L., Coyle, J. T., Fishbach, G. D., Mesulam, M. M., & Sullivan, L. E. (Eds.). (1995). *Memory distortion.* Cambridge: MA: Harvard University Press.

Schaef, A. W. (1981). *Women's reality.* Minneapolis: Winston Press.

Schaefer, C. E., & Briesmeister, J. M. (Eds.). (1989). *Handbook of parent training.* New York: Wiley.

Scheier, M. F., & Carver, C. S. (1987). Dispositional optimism and physical well-being: The influence of generalized expectancies on health. *Journal of Personality, 55,* 169–210.

Scheier, M. F., Weintraub, J. K., & Carver, C. S. (1986). Coping with stress: Divergent strategies of optimists and pessimists. *Journal of Personality and Social Psychology, 51,* 1257–1264.

Schiff, B. B., & Rump, S. A. (1995). Asymmetrical hemispheric activation and emotion: The effects of unilateral forced nostril breathing. *Brain and Cognition, 29,* 217–231.

Schoicket, S. L., Bertelson, A. D., & Lacks, P. (1988). Is sleep hygiene a sufficient treatment for sleep-maintenance insomnia? *Behavior Therapy, 19,* 183–190.

Schuster, R. (1979). Empathy and mindfulness. *Journal of Humanistic Psychology, 19,* 71–77.

Schwartz, B., & Reisberg, D. (1991). *Learning and memory.* New York: Norton.

Schwartz, B., & Robbins, S. J. (1995). *Psychology of learning and behavior* (4th ed.). New York: Norton.

Schwartz, J. M., Stoessel, P. W., Baxter, L. R., Martin, K. M., & Phelps, M. E. (1996). Systematic changes in cerebral glucose metabolic rate after successful behavior modification treatment of obsessive-compulsive disorder. *Archives of General Psychiatry, 53,* 109–113.

Scott, M. (1983). *Kundalini in the physical world.* London: Routledge & Kegan Paul.

Scotton, B. W., Chinen, A. B., & Battista, J. R. (Eds.). (1996). *Textbook of transpersonal psychiatry and psychology.* New York: Basic Books.

Segal, M. H., Campbell, D. T., & Herskovits, M. J. (1966). *The influence of culture on visual perception.* Indianapolis, IN: Bobbs-Merrill.

Segall, Z. V., & Blatt, S. J. (Eds.). (1993). *The self in emotional distress.* New York: Guilford Press.

Seligman, M. E. P. (1970). On the generality of laws of learning. *Psychological Review, 77,* 406–418.

Seligman, M. E. P. (1971). Phobias and preparedness. *Behavior Therapy, 2,* 307–320.

Seligman, M. E. P. (1975). *Learned helplessness.* San Francisco: W. H. Freeman.

Shafranske, E. P. (Ed.). (1996). *Religion and the practice of psychology.* Washington, DC: American Psychological Association.

Shafranske, E. P., & Malony, H. N. (1990). Clinical psychologists' religious and spiritual orientations and their practice of psychotherapy. *Psychotherapy, 27,* 72–78.

Shah, I. (1971a). *The pleasantries of the incredible Mulla Nasrudin.* New York: Dutton.

Shah, I. (1971b). *Wisdom of the idiots.* New York: Dutton.

Shannahoff-Khalsa, D. (1993). The ultradian rhythm of alternating cerebral hemispheric activity. *International Journal of Neuroscience, 70,* 285–298.

Shapiro, D. A., Barkham, M., Reynolds, S., Hardy, G., & Stiles, W. B. (1992). Prescriptive and exploratory psychotherapies: Toward an integration based on the assimilation model. *Journal of Psychotherapy Integration, 4,* 253–272.

Shapiro, D. H. Jr., & Astin, J. A. (1998). *Control therapy.* New York: Wiley.

Shapiro, D. H. Jr., & Walsh, R. N. (Eds.). (1984). *Meditation: Classic and contemporary perspectives.* New York: Aldine.

Sheikh, A. A., & Sheikh, K. S. (Eds.). (1996). *Healing East & West.* New York: Wiley. (1989 title: *Eastern and Western approaches in healing*).

Shephard, I. L. (1970). Limitations and cautions in the gestalt approach. In J. Fagan, & I. L. Shepherd, (Eds.). *Gestalt therapy now.* New York: Harper & Row.

Shields, S. A., Mallory, M. E., & Simon, A. (1989). The Body Awareness Questionnaire: Reliability and validity. *Journal of Personality Assessment, 53,* 802–815.

Silananda, U (1990). *The four foundations of mindfulness.* Boston: Wisdom Publications.

Simon, S., & Simon, S. (1990). *Forgiveness.* New York: Warner Books.

Skinner, B. F. (1974). *About behaviorism.* New York: Knopf.

Skinner, B. F. (1975). The shaping of phylogenic behavior. *Journal of the Experimental Analysis of Behavior, 24,* 117–120.

Sloane, H. N. (1988). *The good kid book.* Champaign, IL: Research Press.

Smith, H. (2000). *The religious significance of entheogenic plants and chemicals.* New York: Tarcher.

Smith, J. C. (1985). *Relaxation dynamics.* Champaign, IL: Research Press.

Snyder, C. R., & Higgins, R. L. (1988). Excuses: Their effective role in the negotiation of reality. *Psychological Bulletin, 104,* 23–35.

Solé-Leris, A. (1986). *Tranquility & insight.* Boston: Shambhala.

Somer, E. (1995). *Food and mood.* New York: Henry Holt.

Soyka, F. (1977). *The ion effect.* New York: Bantam.

Spanos, N. P., Steggles, S., Radtke-Bodorik, H. L., & Rivers, S. M. (1979). Nonanalytic attending, hypnotic susceptibility, and meditators and nonmeditators. *Journal of Abnormal Psychology, 88,* 85–89.

Spiegler, M. D., & Guevremont, D. C. (1998). *Contemporary behavior therapy* (3rd ed.). Pacific Grove, CA: Brooks/Cole.

Squire, L. R., & Kandel, E. R. (2000). *Memory: From mind to molecules.* New York: Scientific American Library.

Staats, A. W. (1996). *Behavior and personality.* New York: Springer.

Stace, W. T. (1960). *The teachings of the mystics.* New York: Mentor Books.

Stallone, J., & Migdal, S. (1991). *Growing sane.* Dallas, PA: Upshur Press.

Starkstein, S. E., Robinson, R. G., & Berthier, M. L. (1992). Post-stroke hallucinatory delusional syndromes. *Neuropsychiatry, Neuropsychology, and Behavioral Neurology, 5,* 114–118.

Stein, K. F., & Markus, H. R. (1994). The organization of the self: An alternative focus for psychopathology and behavior change. *Journal of Psychotherapy Integration, 4,* 317–353.

Stein, K. F., & Markus, H. R. (1996). The role of the self in behavioral change. *Journal of Psychotherapy Integration, 6,* 349–384.

Steketee, G., & White, K. (1990). *When once is not enough.* Oakland, CA: New Harbinger.

Stone, H., & Winkleman, S. (1989). *Embracing our selves: The voice dialogue manual.* San Rafael, CA: New World Library.

Stone, R. (1986). *Polarity therapy* (Vols. 1 & 2). Sebastopol, CA: CRCS Publications.

Storm, H. (1972). *Seven arrows.* New York: Harper & Row.

Strauch, R. (1989). *The reality illusion.* Barrytown, New York: Station Hill Press.

Strayhorn, J. M. Jr. (1977). *Talking it out.* Champaign, IL: Research Press.

Stricker, G., & Gold, J. R. (Eds.). (1993). *Comprehensive handbook of psychotherapy integration.* New York: Plenum Press.

Stuart, R. B. (1983). *Act thin, stay thin.* New York: Jove Publications.

Suinn, R. M. (2001). The terrible twos—anger and anxiety. *American Psychologist, 56,* 27–36.

Suler, J. R. (1993). *Contemporary psychoanalysis and Eastern thought.* Albany: State University of New York Press.

Suls, J. (Ed.). (1982). *Psychological perspectives on the self* (Vol. 1). Hillsdale, NJ: Erlbaum.

Suls, J., & Greenwald, A. G. (Eds.). (1983, 1986). *Psychological perspectives on the self* (Vols. 2 & 3). Hillsdale, NJ: Erlbaum.

Sulzer-Azaroff, B., & Mayer, G. R. (1991). *Behavior analysis for lasting change.* Fort Worth, TX: Holt, Rinehart and Winston.

Suzuki, S. (1970). *Zen mind, beginner's mind.* New York: Weatherhill.

Swann, W. B. Jr. (1997). The trouble with change: Self-verification and allegiance to the self. *Psychological Science, 8,* 177–179.

Szasz, T. S. (1970). *The manufacture of madness.* New York: Harper & Row.

Tanenbaum, J. (1989). *Male & female realities.* Sugar Land, TX: Candle Publishing.

Tannen, D. (1990). *You just don't understand.* New York: Ballatine.

Tannen, D. (1994). *Talking from 9 to 5.* New York: Avon.

Tarpy, R. M. (1997). *Contemporary learning theory and research.* New York: McGraw-Hill.

Tart, C. T. (1972). States of consciousness and state-specific sciences. *Science, 176,* 1203–1210.

Tart, C. T. (1975). *State of consciousness.* New York: Dutton.

Tart, C. T. (1990). Extending mindfulness to everyday life. *Journal of Humanistic Psychology, 30,* 81–106.

Tart, C. T. (Ed.). (1990). *Transpersonal psychologies* (3rd ed.). San Francisco: Harper.

Taylor, S. E. (1989). *Positive illusions.* New York: Basic Books.

Taylor, S. E. (1999). *Health psychology* (4th ed.). Boston: McGraw-Hill.

Taylor, S. E., & Brown, J. D. (1988). Illusion and well-being: A social psychological perspective on mental health. *Psychological Bulletin, 103,* 193–210.

Teri, L., & Wagner, A. (1992). Alzheimer's disease and depression. *Journal of Consulting and Clinical Psychology, 60,* 379–391.

Testa, T. J. (1974). Causal relationships and the acquisition of avoidance responses. *Psychological Review, 81,* 491–505.

Thompson, C. Z. (1981). Will it hurt less if I can control it? A complex answer to a simple question. *Psychological Bulletin, 90,* 89–101.

Thorpe, G. L., & Olson, S. L. (1997). *Behavior therapy* (2nd ed.). Boston: Allyn & Bacon.

Thurman, R. A. E. (1994). *The Tibetan book of the dead.* New York: Bantam Books.

Timmons, B., & Ley, R. (Eds.). (1994). *Behavioral and psychological approaches to breathing disorders.* New York: Plenum Press.

Torgersen, S. (1983). Genetic factors in anxiety disorders. *Archives of General Psychology, 40,* 1085–1088.

Trimble, M. R. (1992). The schizophrenia-like psychosis of epilepsy. *Neuropsychiatry, Neuropsychology, and Behavioral Neurology, 5,* 103–107.

Trungpa, C. (1973). *Cutting through spiritual materialism.* Berkeley, CA: Shambhala.

Turner, J. R., Cardon, L. R., & Hewitt, J. K. (Eds.). (1995). *Behavior genetic approaches in behavioral medicine.* New York: Plenum Press.

Uchino, B. N., Cacioppo, J. T., & Kiecolt-Glaser, J. K. (1996). The relationship between social support and psychological processes: A review with emphasis on underlying mechanisms and implications for health. *Psychological Bulletin, 119,* 488–531.

Uleman, J. S., & Bargh, J. A. (Eds.). (1989). *Unintended thought.* New York: Guilford Press.

Upper, D., & Cautela, J. R. (Eds.). (1979). *Covert conditioning.* Elmsford, NY: Pergamon Press.

Valdez, P., & Mehrabian, A. (1994). Effects of color on emotions. *Journal of Experimental Psychology: General, 123,* 394–409.

van den Hout, M., & Merckelbach, H. (1991). Classical conditioning: Still going strong. *Behavioural Psychotherapy, 19,* 59–79.

van Zomeren, A. H., & Brouwer, W. H. (1994). *Clinical neuropsychology of attention.* New York: Oxford University Press.

Vaughan, F. (1995). *The inward arc* (2nd ed.). Nevada City, CA: Blue Dolphin Press.

Wachtel, P. L. (1977). *Psychoanalysis and behavior therapy.* New York: Basic Books.

Wadden, T. A., & Anderton, C. H. (1982). The clinical use of hypnosis. *Psychological Bulletin, 91,* 215–243.

Wade, J. (1996). *Changes of mind: A holonomic theory of the evolution of consciousness.* Albany: State University of New York Press.

Wallace, B., & Fisher, L. E. (1999). *Consciousness and behavior.* (4th ed.). Boston: Allyn & Bacon.

Walsh, R. (1995). Phenomenological mapping: A method for describing and comparing states of consciousness. *Journal of Transpersonal Psychology, 27,* 25–56.

Walsh, R. (1999). *Essential spirituality.* New York: Wiley.

Walsh, R., & Vaughan, F. (Eds.). (1993). *Paths beyond ego.* Los Angeles: Tarcher.

Wangyal, T. (1998). *The Tibetan yogas of dream and sleep.* Ithaca, NY: Snow Lion.

Ward, C. A. (Ed.). (1989). *Altered states of consciousness and mental health: A cross-cultural perspective.* Newbury Park, CA: Sage.

Washburn, M. (1995). *The ego and the dynamic ground* (2nd ed.). Albany: State University of New York Press.

Watson, D. L., & Tharp, R. G. (1997). *Self-directed behavior* (7th ed.). Pacific Grove, CA: Brooks/Cole.

Watson, J. B. (1913). Psychology as the behaviorist views it. *Psychological Review, 20,* 158–177.

Watts, A. W. (1940). *The meaning of happiness.* New York: Harper & Row.

Webster, J. S., & Scott, R. R. (1988). Behavioral assessment and treatment of the brain-injured patient. In M. Hersen, R. M. Eisler, & P. M. Miller (Eds.), *Progress in behavior modification* (Vol. 22). Newbury Park, CA: Academic Press.

Wegner, D. M., & Pennebaker, J. W. (Eds.). (1993). *Handbook of mental control.* Englewood Cliffs, NJ: Prentice-Hall.

Weil, A. (1973). *The natural mind.* Boston: Houghton-Mifflin.

Weil, G. (1990). Chi-Kung: The Taoist way of cultivating life-force energy, implications for western psychology. In M. G. T. Kwee (Ed.), *Psychotherapy, meditation & health.* London: East-West Publications.

Weisberg, R. W. (1993). *Creativity.* New York: W. H. Freeman.

Weisz, J. R., Rothbaum, F. M., & Blackburn, T. C. (1984). Standing out and standing in: The psychology of control in America and Japan. *American Psychologist, 39,* 955–969.

Wells, A. (1990). Panic disorder in association with relaxation induced anxiety: An attentional training approach to treatment. *Behavior Therapy, 21,* 273–280.

Welwood, J. (1990). *Journey of the heart.* New York: HarperCollins.

Werbach, M. (1991). *Nutritional influences on mental illness.* Tarzana, CA: Third Line Press.

Werbach, M. R. (1988). *Nutritional influence on illness.* Tarzana, CA: Third Line Press.

West, M. A. (Ed.). (1987). *The psychology of meditation.* Oxford, England: Claredon Press.

Westcott, M. R. (1977). Free will: An exercise in metaphysical truth or psychological consequences. *Canadian Psychological Review, 18,* 249–263.

White, J. (Ed.). (1979). *Kundalini, evolution, and enlightenment.* Garden City, NY: Anchor Books.

White, J. (Ed.). (1995). *What is enlightenment?* New York: Paragon House.

White, L., Tursky, B., & Schwartz, G. E. (Eds.). (1985). *Placebo theory, research and mechanisms.* New York: Guilford Press.

Whitmore, D. (1991). *Psychosynthesis counseling in action.* London: Sage.

Wicker, A. W. (1969). Attitudes versus actions: The relationship of verbal and overt behavioral responses to attitude objects. *Journal of Social Issues, 25,* 41–78.

Wigram, T., & DeBacker, J. (Eds.). (1999). *Clinical applications of music therapy in psychiatry.* London: Jessica Kingsley.

Wilber, K. (1977). *The spectrum of consciousness.* Wheaton, IL: Theosophical Publishing House.

Wilber, K. (1980). *The atman project.* Wheaton, IL: Theosophical Publishing House.

Wilber, K. (1983). *Up from eden.* Boulder, CO: Shambhala.

Wilbert K. (1984). *A sociable god.* Bouler, CO: Shambhala.

Wilber, K. (1995). *Sex, ecology, spirituality.* Boston: Shambhala.

Wilber, K. (1996a). *A brief history of everything.* Boston: Shambhala.

Wilber, K. (1996b). *Eye to eye.* (3rd ed.). Boston: Shambhala.

Wilber, K. (2000). *Integral psychology.* Boston: Shambhala.

Williams, J. L. (1973). *Operant learning.* Monterey, CA: Brooks/Cole.

Williams, R. J., & Kalita, D. K. (1977). *A physician's handbook on orthomolecular medicine.* New Canaan, CN: Keats.

Winett, R. A. (1970). Attribution of attitude and behavior change and its relevance to behavior therapy. *Psychological Record, 20,* 17–32.

Winston, S. (1978). *Getting organized.* New York: Warner Books.

Winter, D. A. (1992). *Personal construct psychology in clinical practice.* New York: Routledge, Chapman, & Hall.

Wolman, B. B., & Ullman, M. (Eds.). (1986). *Handbook of states of consciousness.* New York: Van Nostrand Reinhold.

Wong, E. (1997). *The Shambhala guide to Taoism.* Boston: Shambhala.

Worthington, Jr., E. L. Kurusu, T. A., McCullough, M. E., & Sandage, S. J. (1996). Empirical research on religion and psychotherapeutic processes and outcomes: A 10-year review and research prospectus. *Psychological Bulletin, 119,* 448–487.

Wright, P. H. (1977). Perspective on the psychology of self. *Psychological Reports, 40,* 423–436.

Wurtman, J. J. (1988). *Managing your mind and mood through food.* New York: Harper & Row.

Yalom, I. D. (1980). *Existential psychotherapy.* New York: Basic Books.

Yeomans, T. (1974). The pie. *Synthesis, 1,* 97–98.

Zimbardo, P., & Ebbesen, E. B. (1970). *Influencing attitudes and changing behavior.* Reading, MA: Addison-Wesley.

Zweig, C., & Abrams, J. (Eds.). (1990). *Meeting the shadow.* Los Angeles: Tarcher.

Author Index

Subject Index

Acceptance, 73, 81, 120, 133, 145, 169, 171, 173
ADHD/ADD, 93
Advaita-vedanta, 167
Aggression, 23, 33, 37, 38, 39, 57, 80, 118
Aikido, 58
Alcoholism, 33, 54, 158
Allergies, 39, 55
Alternative personal realities, 120
Anapanasati, 52
Anxiety, 33, 34, 39, 40, 48, 49, 53, 55, 57, 91, 100, 101, 134, 136, 146, 159
Applied behavior analysis, 77
Aromatherapy, 47
Art of living, 171
Asana, 5
Assertiveness, 18, 21, 115, 140, 183
Attachments, 99, 101, 103, 114, 115, 130, 135, 147, 169, 183, 184
Attention, 38, 40, 90, 91, 142
Attention disorders, 93
Attentional bias, 93
Attitudes, 78, 79, 80, 89, 97, 103, 119, 122, 133, 171
Attribution, 80, 102, 143, 146
Awakening, 160
Ayurveda, 16, 46, 48, 57, 58, 59

Behavior, 67, 72, 77, 88, 137
Behavior modification, 77, 83, 88, 96, 98, 118, 141
Behavior therapy, 77
Behavioral level, 65, 122, 147, 155, 180, 181
Behavioral medicine, 82
Behaviorism, 67
Behaviors of the mind, 88, 90, 104
Beliefs, 85, 122, 123
Bhakti, 169, 183
Bibliotherapy, 118
Biobehavioral therapy, 45
Biological cycles, 34, 36, 52
Biological level, 29, 67, 73, 81, 95, 148, 155, 180, 181

Bliss, 181
Blood sugar level, 56
Bodywork, 48, 148
Boredom, 104, 150, 183
Breathwork, 50, 53, 62
Buddhism, 60, 61, 71, 72, 79, 80, 89, 95, 96, 100, 107, 121, 124, 132, 134, 143, 144, 163, 169, 173, 183, 184

Catharsis, 49
Chakras, 59, 103, 183
Chi, 58
Chi Kung, 58, 59
Christianity, 15, 89, 101, 188, 144, 157, 169, 171, 183
Circadian rhythms, 35
Clinging, 99, 100, 101
Cognitions, 85
Cognitive behavior therapy, 17, 77, 85
Cognitive science, 86, 91, 111
Cognitive therapy, 17, 85, 94
Color, 46
Communication, 19, 40
Computer models, 86, 87
Concentration, 54, 55, 90, 142, 166
Concentration meditation, 53, 90, 167
Conjunctive psychology, 7, 9, 21, 179, 186
Conjunctive pyramid, 187
Consciousness, 71, 87, 111, 155, 183
   Levels, 124, 162, 167
   States, 120, 184
Consciousness without an object, 163
Control, 146, 147, 148, 166
Craving, 72, 100
Creativity, 103, 183
Cultural differences, 17, 37, 113, 116, 130, 134

Death, 159, 172
Delay of reinforcement, 144
Dependent origination, 71, 100
Depression, 33, 34, 35, 38, 39, 42, 49, 53, 55, 57, 74, 81, 95, 134, 136, 146
Depth perception, 113